STAYING WELL

Why the Good Life Is So Bad for Your Health

Richard E. Ecker

InterVarsity Press
Downers Grove
Illinois 60515

InterVarsity Press is the book-publishing division of Inter-Varsity Christian Fellowship, a student movement active on campus at hundreds of universities, colleges and schools of nursing. For information about local and regional activities, write IVCF, 233 Langdon St., Madison, WI 53703.

Distributed in Canada through InterVarsity Press, 860 Denison St., Unit 3, Markham, Ontario L3R 4H1, Canada.

Cover illustration: Roberta Polfus

ISBN 0-87784-967-6

Printed in the United States of America

Library of Congress Cataloging in Publication Data

Ecker, Richard E., 1930-
    Staying well.

    Includes bibliographical references.
    1. Health.   2. Christian life—1960-   I. Title.
RA776.E193   1984   613   84-4664
ISBN 0-87784-967-6

18	17	16	15	14	13	12	11	10	9	8	7	6	5	4	3	2	1
99	98	97	96	95	94	93	92	91	90	89	88	87	86	85	84

Preface

I set out to write a book showing how the power of God can work wonders in the lives of those who are faithful to him. I found I was saying a lot about achieving a disciplined life. I try to practice what I preach, of course. Otherwise what I've written would have less credibility. I decided to add this preface only after a friend said to me, "You have to remember that not everyone is as disciplined as you are."

Whether or not I am as disciplined as my friend thinks, I want to make something clear at the outset of this book. Having my own life in some degree of order is not in the last analysis my own doing but a consequence of God's grace. God can work wonders. He gives us the ability to change our way of life and to enjoy what happens as we make changes. In that regard, I see myself as a personal witness.

I once weighed twenty-five pounds more than I do now. I was a sedentary person, thoroughly out of condition. I smoked three packs a day and was a fairly heavy drinker. I abused caffeine so severely that it gave me heart rhythm problems. I was so enslaved by stress that I was like a potential time bomb, capable of gross emotional or even physical violence when set off.

But my life has changed. Now I exercise every day without regretting the expenditure of time and effort that it requires. My average heart rate has been lowered by more than fifteen strokes per minute, reducing my heart's annual workload by more than eight million beats. I avoid using substances like alcohol and tobacco that contribute nothing to maintaining health—and I don't feel even one little bit deprived. My outlook on life is more peaceful since I chose to let God do my worrying for me. Those changes have cost me nothing. Indeed, a tremendous personal burden has been lifted from me, and I have never felt better.

So, I look on myself not as being disciplined, but as being re-deemed. Although I will say a lot about personal accountability in the following pages, my primary purpose is not to set a stan-dard for personal discipline. Rather, I want to witness to the availability of God's redeeming love—and to the power of that love to produce change.

1 Life, Death and the Perils of Progress

*S*UPPOSE YOU WERE LIVING SOME EIGHTY YEARS AGO, AT THE TURN of the century. How do you think your life expectancy would compare to the current figures? What would be the primary risks to your life? How would your health compare to what it is now?

The answers to those questions surprise most people. They also tell us something about what contemporary life is doing to people's health. Let's look at the answers and see what kind of progress the twentieth century has brought to our health and life expectancy.[1]

In 1900 in the United States the average life expectancy at birth was about 48 years. Today it's about 74, an impressive increase. But let's look at the data a little more closely. Life expectancy at birth is the average number of years that a newborn can expect to live. In the year 1900 almost 15 per cent of all newborns died in their first year of life. Today infant mortality in the United

States is less than 1.5 per cent, one-tenth what it was then. The biggest single contributor to the increase in overall life expectancy in this century has been a dramatic increase in infant survival.

If we look at the change in life expectancy for people at older ages, we find increases that are much more modest. The first six presidents of the United States lived to an average age of 79.7. The last six who died of natural causes lived to an average age of 73.8. Thousands of years ago, Moses described the span of life in his time: "The years of our life are threescore and ten, or even by reason of strength fourscore" (Ps 90:10).

So we see that people who survive infancy today can't expect a much longer life than people did throughout most of human history. All the medical advances of the twentieth century, all our progress in hygiene and sanitation, all our improvements in nutrition—those things have netted today's adults little in increased life expectancy.

The Twentieth-Century Plague
Why is that? Why have we been able to realize such slight improvement in the span of life when this century has brought so many positive changes in factors that historically have been major causes of early death? We have eliminated plagues and epidemics. We have conquered most of the diseases that struck fear into our ancestors. So why can we expect to live very little longer than they did? The reason is that in our century other causes of mortality have arisen. A new plague is upon us, a twentieth-century plague of major proportions.

At the turn of the century, tuberculosis, typhoid and diphtheria accounted for over 15 per cent of all deaths in the United States. Today, with immunization, antibiotics and improved sanitation, those diseases cause less than one-tenth of 1 per cent of all U.S. mortality. On the other hand, deaths from cardiovascular problems (major diseases of the heart and circulation) increased by almost 50 per cent in the first half of this century. And although the rate has declined slightly in recent years, those diseases still constitute the largest single cause of mortality in the United States: over 1 million deaths per year—half of the total from all causes.

The death rate from cancer has tripled since the turn of the century. Although deaths from cirrhosis of the liver declined significantly when prohibition was instituted in the United States, the mortality rate from that disease has doubled since repeal of prohibition in 1932. The death rate from diabetes has also increased steadily in this century. Statistics on diabetes mortality are somewhat confused, however, because that disease has so many complications (such as heart and kidney disease) which are frequently listed as the primary cause of death.

Thus mortality in the twentieth century has been affected both by elimination of the vast majority of the historical causes of early death and by their replacement with a new group of diseases that were relatively rare in earlier history. Yet mortality is not the most telling statistic with which to evaluate our health status.

One important accomplishment of medicine in the past few decades is the ability to delay fatality in people who suffer life-shortening diseases. For example, a decline in U.S. mortality from heart disease in the past ten to fifteen years has been due, at least in part, to improvements in the scope and quality of emergency medicine. Because we have many more trained paraprofessionals and well-equipped trauma centers today, people who suffer heart attacks have a much better chance of immediate survival. Further, improvements in rehabilitation medicine give those patients a better chance of continued survival.

Still, it is important to understand that people in this country continue to suffer heart attacks with alarming frequency. We have not developed healthier hearts in the last decade—we have learned how to survive longer with unhealthy ones.

Today about 43 million Americans have some form of cardio-vascular disease.[2] This year, some one and a half million Americans will suffer heart attacks, of whom one-third will not survive the year. Over 300,000 Americans have lung cancer, about one-third of whom won't survive beyond twelve months. And, by the end of the same year, there will be 135,000 new lung-cancer victims to take their place. Diabetes now affects an estimated 11 million Americans and, according to a recent actuarial study, its incidence in the population is doubling every fifteen years. That study goes on to say, "The average American born today has a better than one in five chance of developing diabetes."[3]

The Risks of Progress

Why are these degenerative, life-shortening diseases so prevalent in our society? Why do they continue to increase at almost epidemic rates? Why have we become victimized by diseases that were once so rare and that are still uncommon among primitive societies? The answer is in the *choices* we make. We are suffering illness, disability and death unnecessarily because of the way we choose to live.

Progress has granted us a multitude of lifestyle options. For most of us, dietary alternatives are almost unlimited—as are our opportunities to avoid physical activity. Further, powerful drugs known or suspected to be harmful are distributed legally through normal channels of commerce. And not the least of the fruits of progress has been an increased exposure to unsettling change, creating an environment of uncertainty that prompts us to react with stress. Regrettably such "progress" has not been accompanied by an increased public understanding of the risks that accompany each choice. As a result, decisions are often made in ignorance. As we have seen, the health consequences of such ignorance have been, and continue to be, devastating.

My goals in the following chapters are to explore the tremendous influence our choice of lifestyle has on health, well-being and life expectancy; to demonstrate some specific kinds of lifestyle changes we can make to avoid unnecessary disease; to assess such changes in the light of commitment to responsible Christian stewardship; and to provide a scripturally sound strategy for implementing desirable changes.

2 Making Choices

*PARTICIPANTS IN A WEIGHT-MANAGEMENT CLASS WERE DISCUSS-*ing what had contributed to their overweight problem and what stood in the way of the solution. One man volunteered that his biggest obstacle was too much of "the good life." That statement did more than pinpoint one individual's stumbling block on the path to good health. It also summarized the single most important health problem in Western society today.

The Good Life—Why Is It So Bad for Health?
Four basic categories of choice in lifestyle influence our health and can become contributing causes of degenerative disease: (1) diet, (2) substance abuse, (3) physical inactivity and (4) stress. Later chapters will discuss each influence in detail. Here I will consider them only in a general way to get an overview of how lifestyle is related to health. First, though, let me point out that

even today we start off life with a clean bill of health. The human body is naturally disposed to good health. With few exceptions, we are well when we enter this world, and we have full potential to maintain that state for a long life.

In this chapter I want to look at the health potential of the human body as it begins life and what is required to maintain that health. I will also consider the development of modern societies and how the changes in the choices people make have influenced modern lifestyles. Finally, I will discuss how those lifestyles work to destroy the physical attributes that are essential to health.

At birth, or reasonably soon thereafter, the human body is equipped with most of the characteristics it will need to adapt physiologically (that is, in its internal chemistry) to its environment. Of course the newborn is not socially self-sufficient, but it can perform most of the physiological processes that will sustain it throughout life. It can digest food and distribute the products of digestion to the parts of the body where they are needed for energy and growth. It can maintain a remarkable constancy in body temperature and internal chemistry. It can purge itself of many potentially toxic substances. It can fight off infectious agents and, in the process, enhance its defenses against a subsequent invasion.

Its most fundamental attribute is adaptability. In the human being, as in all living creatures, stability is the key to survival. Yet the world is fundamentally an unstable place to be in. The only way to survive in such a changeable environment is to be well equipped to adapt. To insure survival, we are born with a variety of mechanisms for maintaining physiological stability. Those mechanisms, however, are not indestructible. If they are consistently abused, they may ultimately break down. In fact, our adaptation mechanisms are the primary victims of the good life.

As we develop and mature, we increase in strength, coordination, intelligence and awareness. Yet we acquire little additional capability for physiological adaptation. We do, however, acquire one new dimension in adaptability: the emotional. This has great survival value. It helps an individual's physical and intellectual achievements relate constructively with the realities of life. Yet the mechanisms for emotional adaptation are themselves susceptible both to flaws in their formation and to abuse in their application.

When people have few options to choose from in electing a way of life, they have little responsibility for their choices. If the only options they have allow nothing but potentially damaging choices, they become genuine victims of their circumstances. At the other extreme are people whose options permit only beneficial choices. These people may never be aware that the outcome of their choosing is really a gift of their circumstances. When choices are abundant, however, options are usually both beneficial and potentially harmful. In this case the individual bears much greater responsibility for the consequences—whether good or bad.

At the beginning of the twentieth century, a typical North American had few lifestyle options. At that time, 52 per cent of the U.S. population lived on farms.[1] Rural life was characterized by hard physical labor, relative isolation from the rest of the culture and a diet dictated by what was locally available. For the rest of the population, physical labor was the basis of almost all employment, since few labor-saving conveniences were available. Outside the rural areas, dietary options were limited by slow transportation and undependable storage. There was little spare time. Opportunity for travel was limited. Family relationships were stronger and more permanent. Values were more universally accepted and more clearly defined. And restrictions imposed by conditions of the time were less likely to be viewed as personally threatening. Most people built their lifestyles on the few choices available to them. Basically these choices were good for health, or at least not so damaging as many choices made today.

Perhaps the most fundamental change in lifestyle in this century has been a marked reduction in physical activity. The good life today is synonymous with the avoidance of physical exertion. Automobiles, convenient parking, elevators, escalators and labor savers of all kinds make it almost unnecessary for us to lift a finger either to do our jobs or to enjoy our leisure. But for most of us, this decrease in physical activity has not been accompanied by a comparable decrease in calorie intake. As a result, over one-third of the adult population today is enough overweight that their weight contributes significantly to their risk of disease.[2] Physical exertion is one mechanism that helps maintain the body's health. When that mechanism is missing, our ability to adapt is diminished and our bodies become more susceptible to other negative lifestyle influences.

Another significant lifestyle change has accompanied the development of Western culture in the twentieth century—the way we eat. Our almost unlimited dietary choices today are seldom made on the basis of what is best for preserving our health. The good life has made *taste, convenience* and *appearance* the big three in food selection. As a result, our diets have become a major contributor to our declining health.

There is no question that the use of potentially harmful drugs has increased substantially in this century. In 1900, for example, 51 cigarettes per person were produced in the United States. In 1970 the number had increased to 2,743 per person. Although some of that increase is obviously the result of increased exports, and although "roll-your-own" cigarettes were more popular in the early years of this century, a more than fiftyfold increase in per capita cigarette production clearly indicates a dramatic in-

crease in smoking. The health consequences of that major lifestyle change can be found in a currently exploding incidence of
lung cancer among Americans. And, although alcohol consumption has not increased so dramatically, its effects are no less dis-
turbing. Over 5 per cent of the population, more than one in
every twenty Americans, is presently alcoholic.[3] For many others
alcohol use is a significant health deterrent.

Another significant factor in modern society increasing the
risk of disease is stress. Although stress is difficult to measure,
the majority of us would undoubtedly agree that it is a greater
problem today than it has been in the past. Like other risk factors, stress in America has grown with the good life. Improvement in life's social and economic qualities has put increased
demands on the individual. The pressures of these demands
create uncertainty, and uncertainty breeds stress. A prime consequence of uncontrolled stress is a disintegration in emotional
adaptability. Such a breakdown can overload the mechanisms of
physical adaptation, virtually guaranteeing some degenerative
physical effects.

The good life is bad for health because its choices overwhelm
the ability of our inborn system to maintain good health. From
that perspective, such a life is not really good at all. Although it
has many inviting short-term rewards, the good life carries the
seeds of destruction. Other alternatives, however, do offer hope
for something better: a long and healthy life. In the final analysis,
we have a choice.

Heredity and Environment
So far I have barely mentioned heredity. That is not because I
consider heredity an unimportant factor in the tendency of some
people to develop degenerative diseases. Considering all the evidence, I believe that environment (lifestyle, in particular) is far
more crucial. For some people, that conclusion should be a

source of considerable hope. After all, though we cannot control our inheritance, we can usually control our lifestyles.

What about those negative environmental influences we have almost no control over—such as air and water pollution, chemical contamination of foods and the possible toxicity of food and water additives? For some people, such influences may be extremely significant. Again, however, on the basis of the evidence, I conclude that the health threat currently constituted by those influences is nowhere near the proportions of the threat caused by elective lifestyles.

Let us put the matter of heredity into an understandable perspective. There is no doubt that cardiovascular disease, diabetes and even alcoholism all tend to occur more frequently in certain families. Unquestionably, susceptibility to certain degenerative diseases can be inherited. But what is a person susceptible to when he or she inherits a tendency to a degenerative disease? Does the body simply degenerate? Is that person irrevocably fated at birth to disease in later life? Certainly there is a body of opinion that holds that view. In general, I do not. As I pointed out earlier, I believe that, with few exceptions, the human body is naturally disposed toward good health. I believe that the destruction of that healthful disposition is an active process, contributed to primarily by each individual's lifestyle. All that a high-risk person inherits is a susceptibility to the abusive effects of certain lifestyles. If abuses do not occur, inherited susceptibility is of little consequence.

To illustrate, imagine that you have been given a valuable cut-glass goblet. Although it is very fragile, the goblet is perfectly serviceable and, if you care for it gently, you can use it indefinitely. If you treat it roughly, however, the chances are that it will break and become useless. On the other hand, suppose that you were given an equally valuable silver goblet. That sturdy vessel can endure a great deal of abuse without breaking. Even if you treat it roughly, it will probably still serve you indefinitely.

The two goblets represent the extremes of inherited tendencies for degenerative disease. Some people inherit a high risk of damage from lifestyle abuse. Others inherit a low risk. Most of us are somewhere in between. Our tendencies do not destine us to disease—they merely decrease our resistance to the good life.

We have two alternatives to avoid the risks of life-shortening degenerative diseases: either we are born with a high resistance to health-abusive lifestyles, or we must avoid those lifestyles. Since most of us don't know until it's too late whether or not we qualify for the first alternative, the second is the only sure way to lower our risk.

While I said earlier that most people are born with a natural tendency toward health, I acknowledged that there were exceptions. Let us consider those exceptions to illustrate even more graphically the value of a controlled lifestyle. Individuals with certain "inborn errors of metabolism" are deficient from birth in their ability to establish the internal chemical stability required to maintain health. Without careful regulation of lifestyle they find it difficult, sometimes impossible, to survive. Yet by carefully controlling their lifestyles, they can often lead nearly normal lives.

One example of such an inborn deficiency is a condition called phenylketonuria, commonly abbreviated as PKU. PKU is characterized by the body's inability to utilize certain amino acids found in most dietary proteins. If such proteins are included in the diet, an individual with PKU will suffer severe mental retardation. If the proteins are avoided, retardation effects can be significantly reduced. Nowadays, newborns are routinely tested for PKU and, if found to possess the trait, are placed on diets that avoid the offending proteins. In other words, their lifestyles are adjusted to prevent abuses to their impaired metabolic capabilities.

So, whether we inherit some tendency to higher life-risk or a full-blown metabolic deficiency, it is our environment, determined largely by our lifestyles, that causes the trait to be expressed in disease—or suppressed into harmlessness. Our goal, then, is to choose our lifestyles wisely.

3 The Stewardship of Health

*F*OR CHRISTIANS, CHOOSING A LIFESTYLE IS IMPORTANT FOR MORE reasons than the physical and emotional consequences. We are accountable to God for the wise management of resources entrusted to our care. Our choices are the way we exercise Christian stewardship.

"That Your Days May Be Prolonged"

What is our responsibility for the stewardship of health? Two points seem clear from Scripture. First, although biblical references to the stewardship of health are seldom specific, God expects his people to meet this responsibility as diligently as all our other stewardship obligations. Second, since the specific references are limited primarily to Old Testament ceremonial regulations, God must expect Christians to exercise personal judgment in our stewardship of health. Our behavior must satisfy his overall purpose in giving us life in the first place. We must therefore find out what a biblical understanding of that purpose is.

Can we assume, first of all, that God wants us to live long and healthy lives? I find compelling support for that view in Scripture. Mortal life, although short when measured by the standards of eternity, is precious to God. One of his purposes in giving the commandments was "that your days may be prolonged" (Deut 6:2). Through Solomon he reiterated his concern for the value of mortal life. "The fear of the LORD is the beginning of wisdom, and the knowledge of the Holy One is insight. For by me *your days will be multiplied, and years will be added to your life*" (Prov 9:10-11).

In his earthly ministry, Jesus healed the sick. He gave a chance for prolonged life to many who were hopelessly afflicted. He wept when his friend Lazarus died and brought him back to life (Jn 11:17-44). Jesus sustained people with food when they were hungry (Mt 14:15-21; 15:32-38). He told his followers that when they took care of the bodily needs of his earthly "brethren" they would be honoring him (Mt 25:34-45). Long life is a biblically sound goal.

If God gives us the potential for good health, what obligation do we have to maintain our health? Probably the most familiar biblical reference about our bodies is this statement by the apostle Paul: "Do you not know that your body is a temple of the Holy Spirit within you, which you have from God? You are not your own; you were bought with a price. *So glorify God in your body*" (1 Cor 6:19-20). How do we glorify God in our bodies? We must take our cues from other references in Scripture about the general obligations of Christian stewardship.

Jesus said, "Every one to whom much is given, of him will much be required" (Lk 12:48). Jesus hammered home the obligations of stewardship in a number of his parables, making it clear that God's gifts are not to be neglected, abandoned or wasted.

They are all to be used, and used wisely, applying good judgment about God's intentions whenever specific instructions are lacking. The parables also make a final point: when our mortal service to the Creator is completed, we will be called to account for our stewardship.

Consider God's gift of health. As stewards, we are expected to preserve that gift with every resource available to us. Health is always subject to assault by factors over which we have no control. Yet we *can* control most of the influences that today cause degenerative disease and premature death. Responsible stewardship of health means choosing to exercise that control.

The Narrow Gate, the Hard Choice

Perhaps Jesus' simplest and most direct teaching about making choices came at the end of the Sermon on the Mount: "Enter by the narrow gate; for the gate is wide and the way is easy, that leads to destruction, and those who enter it are many. For the gate is narrow and the way is hard, that leads to life, and those who find it are few" (Mt 7:13-14). In that statement Jesus articulated a life principle most of us know well: constructive choices in life are often difficult to make; easy choices often lead to destructive outcomes.

That principle is usually applied to moral decisions and eternal outcomes. But I find no reason to assume that Jesus meant to be restrictive here in speaking of "life" or "destruction." While we live out our mortal lives, our Lord is as concerned for our physical well-being as he is for our spiritual welfare. The wide and narrow gates are not moral abstractions—they represent the kinds of options with which people are confronted daily.

Perhaps it is the starkness of Jesus' words that makes us reluctant to apply them to everyday situations. We are willing to picture ultimate questions of good and evil, of heaven and hell, in contrasting extremes of "black and white." But in this present life, many will say, our choices are seldom so clear-cut—there are many "gray areas." That kind of argument may be helpful to keep us from being judgmental about a particular choice made by another individual. But I believe it is wrong to seek comfort in our own exercise of stewardship by trying to compromise Jesus' teachings on the matter of choice. His followers have no alternative to responsible stewardship—in all areas of life.

Hope abounds in Jesus' teachings, but that hope is not to be based on any compromise of the requirements set down for his stewards. Those requirements—"the narrow way"—are hard and Jesus seems not to give an inch in his expectation that they should be followed. Our hope comes not from lessening our obligations but from God's firm promise of continued love and forgiveness even if we fail to meet those obligations.

I will have much more to say about Christian hope later on. Here, however, I need to establish a perspective on its real source because, without sounding like a "doomsayer," I intend to present a factual case for our *failure* as stewards of health. Of course (and here I speak from considerable personal experience), failure is usually the first step in the process of Christian growth. Out of failure comes awareness. Out of awareness comes a desire to change (that is, repentance). Through repentance comes God's forgiving grace. And through grace comes the strength to obey, endure and succeed.

My purpose in presenting the realities of failure is to lay a foundation for change. I want to provide a witness to the one basis for hope that can lead to positive change for everyone who truly wants it. I may sound harsh when I speak of failure, but I have no desire to pass judgment on any individuals who fail. Admittedly the realities are often unpleasant. But I cannot be true to my purpose without focusing on them and on their consequences.

For example, being overweight contributes significantly to several life-shortening diseases. One of the harsh realities of our health mismanagement is the fact that one-third of the American population is overweight. It is also a fact that this high proportion of overweight exists primarily because of our eating habits. Another harsh reality is the fact that 95 per cent of all people who try to lose weight fail to do so.

As unpleasant as these realities may be, they are realities. I've worked with enough overweight people, however, to know that it can be a tremendous personal burden. Frequently it is a source of intense suffering, amplified by a feeling of powerlessness. In no way do I intend to make light of that suffering. On the other hand, the suffering does not alter the facts. Like all of the degenerative conditions I will be discussing, overweight exists largely by choice and is eliminated by choice. It would be a disservice to overweight readers to gloss over that reality in order to avoid treading on personal sensitivities. The realities must be accurately identified and accepted for what they are if change is to take place.

So we begin by acknowledging that it is a Christian's responsibility in life to make some hard choices. Yet we also affirm that believers have available an inexhaustible source of power to help us make those hard choices. Jesus promised to stand with us in times of need, to be a source of strength when things seem humanly impossible: "If you abide in me, and my words abide in you, ask whatever you will, and it shall be done for you" (Jn 15:7). Paul also assured us, "No temptation has overtaken you that is not common to man. God is faithful, and he will not let you be tempted beyond your strength, but with the temptation will also provide the way of escape, that you may be able to endure it" (1 Cor 10:13).

God requires that we make hard choices. But he also guarantees that, when the time comes to choose, he will provide whatever resources we need to make the right decisions.

4 Nutrition, Health and Disease

*W*HAT NUTRITIONAL DEFICIENCY IS MOST SIGNIFICANT IN THE American diet? If you asked an average group of consumers that question, the most frequent answer would probably be vitamins. The tremendous volume of vitamin supplements currently sold in this country clearly indicates such an opinion. Further, the amount of advertising devoted to vitamins and vitamin-fortified products shows that it is profitable for certain industries to promote that viewpoint among consumers. The fact is, however, that vitamin deficiency is not a real health problem for the vast majority of us. Probably only a small fraction of all the vitamins distributed in this country actually contributes to anyone's health or longevity.

The Vitamin Culture
Some efforts to peddle unnecessary vitamins to uninformed con-

sumers border on the immoral. Take the so-called "stress formula" vitamins, for example. Vitamins have absolutely no value either for preventing the occurrence of stress or for overcoming any of the physical effects that stress produces in the body. Yet vitamin preparations with the word *stress* in their labeling clearly imply that the vitamins will prevent or ameliorate the experience of stress. Obviously, that is the reason most people buy such preparations. In that respect, the labeling is patently misleading. Stress formula vitamins are nothing but regular vitamin supplements with an inappropriate name.

The main reason that vitamin supplements are so popular, in my opinion, is that they are convenient to use. If your lifestyle leaves you in a state of diminished health, or if stress has made your life less tolerable, you can take a vitamin pill. It's an easy choice. It doesn't require that you confront the lifestyle choices that are actually responsible for your diminished health or unwanted stress.

The most damaging aspect of our participation in our "vitamin culture" is that public attention is shifted away from real dietary factors associated with degenerative disease. Vitamin deficiency disease is virtually unheard of in modern Western society. Even what vitamin cultists describe as "marginal deficiencies" have not been shown to have any measurable effect on health or life expectancy. For the vast majority of us, the choice to take supplemental vitamins won't add a day to our lives. Other dietary choices, however, may take years from our lives.

This is not to say that supplemental vitamins are never necessary. Sometimes an individual's minimum need for a particular vitamin (or other essential nutrient) cannot be obtained in the diet that is available or required. My intention here is not to suggest that such circumstances never occur, only that they are not common in our culture.

Among degenerative conditions caused or contributed to by

dietary factors, three are of particular importance because they can be so destructive. They are (1) *overweight*, (2) *cardiovascular disease* and (3) *diabetes*. The three conditions are interrelated. They have some common physiological origins and express some common degenerative effects. Another serious condition, (4) *lower bowel disease*, will also be considered because of its clear association with diet and its increasing prevalence in modern Western society. For each condition I will examine what is known about the role of diet as a causative factor.

Overweight

Overweight is a health problem of major proportions. It affects the health potential of at least one-third of our population. It is considered to be a significant risk factor in a number of degenerative diseases, including cardiovascular disease, gallbladder disease, diabetes and uterine cancer.[1] The word *overweight* is used here rather than *obesity* because the term *obese* is usually applied only to that segment of overweight people who are grossly above normal body weight.

There is no universally accepted standard for determining at what point an overweight person becomes obese. Commonly, people are classified as obese when their weight exceeds by over 20 per cent the weight considered ideal for their height. Whatever the definition of obesity, however, it is incorrect to assume that excess body weight becomes a health risk only after a person qualifies for that definition. Excess body weight contributes to health risk at *any* level above normal. Hence I refer to the risk factor as overweight.

Because overweight is so common, it is often overlooked as a health problem. People tend to accept it as a normal part of the human condition, preferring to believe that they have no personal responsibility for their excess weight, that it was dealt to them by fate. The fantasy that we are "victims" of overweight

---

may be personally comforting, but the facts tell a different story. Very few people are overweight because of factors beyond their own control. With a handful of exceptions, the occurrence of overweight in modern society has resulted because individuals have followed eating patterns that promote the accumulation of excess body fat. They remain overweight because such patterns remain a part of their lifestyles. Of course, we have to eat to obtain the nutrients our bodies need to function properly. For example, the daily diet provides the essential building materials that are required for the growth, repair and replacement of tissues. Only a small fraction of total dietary intake is used for that purpose, however.

The body's most overwhelming requirement is for energy. Over 95 per cent of the food an adult human consumes is used as fuel to produce energy. (Foods are commonly rated by the calories they provide, and a calorie is a measure of energy.) In an average person, most of the energy used in a typical day is devoted to what is called *basal metabolism,* the basic bodily functions required for life: maintenance of body temperature and operation of the brain and heart, to name just a few. Because such functions continue constantly and because they have a very high requirement for energy, a constant supply of fuel must always be available.

But because we don't eat constantly, the body also has to have mechanisms to store fuel in times of plenty (right after meals) and to recall that fuel in times of famine (between meals). This capacity for fuel storage and recovery is part of the process of physiological adaptation I described earlier as the key element in the body's inborn tendency toward good health. The storage process assures stability in the availability of fuel for normal metabolic activity.

The human body uses two kinds of substances as its primary fuels, carbohydrate and fat. Protein, the third of the three major nutrients, is important primarily as a material for building body structures. It is used as a fuel only when it is overabundant in the diet or when it is the only substance available to meet immediate energy needs. Carbohydrate and fat are both stored in the body in fuel reservoirs. Protein exists in the body only in essential tissue structures—for example, in blood components, muscles and other cells.

The body's carbohydrate stores are maintained in three locations: in muscle cells in the form of muscle glycogen; in the liver as liver glycogen; and in the blood as blood sugar. When food containing carbohydrates (that is, those composed of sugars and starches) are digested, simple sugars are released and picked up in the blood where they become blood sugar. The blood then carries that sugar to various parts of the body either to be used directly as fuel by the tissues or to be stored away for use later.

Except for the muscles and liver, none of the tissues of the body can store fuel. As a result, they have to depend on the blood to provide a constant supply. In most cases, that fuel can be either carbohydrate (sugar) or fat. In one case, the brain, only blood sugar can be used as fuel. Thus, in a sense, the blood also serves as an essential reservoir for carbohydrate fuel.

Stored carbohydrate fuel serves different functions depending on its storage site. Muscle glycogen is used only to provide energy for the muscle cells in which it is stored. Liver glycogen is a blood-sugar reserve, helping to maintain a constant availability of fuel primarily for the brain. The total storage capacity of the liver and blood for carbohydrate fuel is, however, quite limited. Without a regular resupply from the diet, those reserves are exhausted in a matter of hours.

Fat is the primary storage form for excess calories from the diet. Fat has, in fact, all the attributes of an ideal storage fuel. First, virtually anything you eat will be converted by your body into fat if not needed immediately for some specific function.

Second, fat has a very high calorie density; that is, it can store a lot of calories in a small volume. Third, it can be used as a fuel by most of the tissues of the body and, in cases of extended starvation, it can be converted into a form that even the brain can use for fuel. Fourth, the body's capacity for fat storage is almost unlimited. If you have had a problem with overweight, this property may seem anything but ideal. Just remember, however, the body's interest is internal stability, not appearance. The purpose of our capacity to store fat is survival.

Those facts, then, bring us to the heart of the problem of overweight as a disease and as a contributor to disease. The mechanism by which the body stores excess calories as body fat can be considered a survival process simply because some accumulation of body fat is a useful guard against future starvation. The prime purpose for fat storage is to enable the body to function in the face of dietary excess, an instability to which the body must necessarily adapt. That kind of adaptation does not serve any essential physiological need. It merely eliminates the instability—disposes of the excess. Fat in the tissues is in a sense the body's garbage dump. You would not function well with your house full of refuse; your body feels the same way when it is full of excess calories.

Depositing excessive fat in the tissues is a degenerative process. It is an abnormality that can interfere with a variety of the body's normal functions. It can diminish physical mobility and endurance. It causes fat deposits in the walls of blood vessels (which we will discuss later). It also promotes malfunctions in other adaptation processes. For example, overweight people tend to have very abnormal insulin responses compared to people of normal weight.[2] Such effects greatly increase the susceptibility of an overweight person to other degenerative diseases. Thus, once the body's ability to adapt to its circumstances has been pushed beyond its intended limits, the consequences can easily be compounded into serious disease.

One other consideration of overweight needs to be discussed here because it, too, can be a cause of degenerative effects: weight-loss dieting. As pointed out earlier, weight-loss dieting has a poor record of success. Few people are willing to make the hard choices necessary for healthy weight loss. When it comes to losing weight, most opt for the easy choices. That is why diet books sell so well, and why supermarket tabloids and women's magazines seldom put out an issue without offering a new diet, promising fast results. If weight-loss dieting were easy, it would be more than five per cent successful, but lack of success isn't the only problem. Another is the degenerative effects created by many of the popular weight-loss plans.

Many people base their approach to weight management on the erroneous assumption that weight loss is the exact reverse of weight gain—that if you gain weight by eating, then the best way to lose weight is by starving. A better understanding of physiology would help put that myth to rest. The basic principle behind weight-loss dieting is simple: when calorie intake is reduced below what is required to meet the body's daily energy demand, the resulting fuel deficit will be made up from stores of body fat. Not all of the body's energy requirements, however, can be satisfied by using fat as fuel. As mentioned earlier, certain tissues, those of the brain in particular, have specific requirements for carbohydrate fuel (blood sugar). Those requirements are the first priority in the process of fuel supply, and they are continuous.

Thus, proper energy economy in the body depends on more than *how much* one eats. It also depends on *what* and *when*. The minimum energy demand of the brain in an average person translates into about three and a half grams of blood sugar per hour. That is a continuous minimum fuel requirement that *must* be satisfied. Many other tissues, however, will use blood sugar preferentially when it is available, putting them in constant competition with the brain for that essential fuel.

What do you suppose will happen if the dietary supply of carbohydrate is insufficient to provide your brain's minimum need for fuel in such a competitive environment? One or more of several things will happen.

As the supply of sugar in the blood decreases, the body will call on its glycogen reserves in the liver to make up the deficit. If that reserve is not adequate, it will convert protein from the diet into blood sugar, provided such dietary protein is immediately available. If not, the body will destroy its own essential tissues to obtain protein to convert into blood sugar. Whatever has to be done, the brain's need for fuel will be satisfied.

Diets that minimize the total intake of carbohydrates promote depletion of liver glycogen reserves and lead to conversion of proteins into blood sugar. That conversion process is highly inefficient. So, in some people, even reducing diets that are high in protein may still be inadequate to meet the body's need both for tissue synthesis and for blood sugar. The net result will then be a loss of lean body tissue rather than loss of fat. When that happens weight loss may be substantial, but with little elimination of body fat.

That kind of weight loss is the basis of most of the "quickie" diets. It is not a healthy process. Rather it is itself a degenerative process which, in some extreme cases, has led to death.

There is no easy way to get rid of accumulated body fat. To lose weight safely and effectively, body-fat reserves have to be integrated cautiously into the total energy economy of the body. Some practical strategies to accomplish that goal will be discussed in the next chapter.

Finally, I would like to make a brief comment about fasting. Considering the statements just made, outlining our body's constant need for dietary fuel to avoid degenerative effects in the tissues, I believe strongly that fasting is a poor strategy for losing weight. On what I consider to be sound physiological grounds, I also reject the idea that fasting in any way purges the body of "accumulated poisons." I acknowledge and endorse, however, the scriptural admonition for Christian believers to fast as a means of spiritual renewal and as an adjunct to prayer.

Throughout history, the people of God have abstained from food for periods of time to humble themselves before him and petition for his mercy. As I have tried to emphasize, the human body is a remarkably adaptable organism. Within its adaptive capabilities, it can easily adjust to such temporary deprivation. At the end of a fast it will readjust rapidly to make up for any deficiencies experienced during the deprivation. Fasting for reasonable periods of time cannot be considered a basically harmful practice. Its effects are seldom permanent. Of course, the same can be said for fasting as a strategy in weight loss. Its results are seldom permanent.

Cardiovascular Disease

Cardiovascular disease (CVD) is generally the result of a degenerative condition in the blood vessels. That condition, called atherosclerosis, is characterized by a thickening of the vessel walls from deposits of fat and cholesterol. The role of the diet as a possible factor in that process has been a matter of speculation in the medical community for many years. After a century and a half of continued research and scientific debate, it has yet to be definitely established.

We know that elevated serum concentrations of certain fat derivatives (particularly cholesterol) greatly increase the risk of an individual for CVD, and it is generally agreed that such high serum cholesterol levels constitute a prime cause of atherosclerosis. It is also known that, in experimental animals (and in some people), higher proportions of fat, especially saturated fat, and of cholesterol in the diet contribute to elevated serum cholesterol.[3] What is not clear at present is whether dietary fat can be considered a significant CVD risk factor for all people. The current wisdom in medical practice and public education is to recommend a restricted intake of fat and cholesterol for everyone.[4] Considering the fact that only minimal amounts of dietary fat are needed to maintain human health, that recommendation appears sound.

Not all authorities, however, agree that fat and cholesterol are the primary dietary factors contributing to the risk for CVD. A significant body of evidence implicates dietary sugar as a more significant contributing factor.[5] Among several convincing lines of evidence are experiments showing that when people moved from a more rural to a more urban living environment, CVD among them increased dramatically within a few years.[6] The people studied had no difference in fat intake in the two settings, and saturated fat intake was actually greater among those with the lower incidence of CVD. On the other hand, refined sugar intake increased more than tenfold among those who moved to the cities.[7] Of course, diet was not the only change experienced by the people who moved. They became more overweight and, although we have no direct evidence, it is likely that their experience of stress increased when they moved into the urban setting. Overweight and stress are both believed to be factors contributing to the risk of developing CVD. Of greater significance is the fact that among the people studied, within twenty-five years following their change in lifestyle, the incidence of diabetes increased by some fortyfold.[8] Diabetes is a major factor contributing to one's risk of developing CVD. Thus it is very possible that the two diseases share some common origins stemming from the diet. After I discuss the role of diet in the occurrence of diabetes, I will return briefly to CVD and try to put any common cause-and-effect relationships into perspective.

One other significant dietary factor in the cause of cardiovascular disease is sodium. Of the almost 43 million current CVD patients in the United States, over 85 per cent suffer from hypertension (high blood pressure). That degenerative condition is a prime contributor to the more fatal forms of CVD, such as heart attack and stroke. Evidence continues to accumulate that dietary sodium is a major contributor in the cause and aggravation of hypertension. The average American consumes almost 5,000 milligrams of sodium in a typical day, over twenty times what is required to meet the body's minimum need for the mineral.[9] By far the largest sources of sodium in the typical American diet are from fast-food items, salt added at the table and in prepared foods (particularly canned foods—vegetables, meats and specialty items).

Almost from birth, we cultivate a taste for excess salt. As a result, adults are so dulled to the flavor of sodium chloride that only excessive amounts of it can satisfy their need for its taste. To add salt is an easy choice. The hard choice is to change to a new way of life, learning to appreciate the taste of foods with a minimum of salt. The easy choice has helped give some 37 million Americans high blood pressure. The only way to turn that situation around is for us to start making the hard choice.

Diabetes

Diabetes is a disease characterized by an impaired ability to use carbohydrates and excessive sugar in the blood. Diabetes is an incurable disease, although many of its symptoms can be controlled through careful medical management. It is usually believed to be inherited. But that assumption is for the most part incorrect.

This complex disease expresses itself in a variety of ways. The most severe type is what has traditionally been referred to as "juvenile-onset" diabetes, now called "insulin-dependent" diabetes. Patients who have it typically require insulin-injection therapy from onset. Most people affected with this form of the disease are less than twenty years of age at the time of onset. Insulin-dependent diabetes comprises less than 5 per cent of all new cases.

The more common form has traditionally been known as "adult-onset" diabetes. Now it is called "noninsulin-dependent" diabetes because many patients who have it can be controlled without the use of insulin therapy. It predominately affects people over the age of forty-five. In this group almost one in every ten Americans now has the disease. I will use the traditional names for the two conditions in this discussion.

Juvenile-onset diabetes is an inherited disease. Lifestyle is not a significant factor in its occurrence. By contrast, the adult-onset form, which is often erroneously thought to be hereditary, is caused primarily by lifestyle. Without getting overly technical, I want to discuss the origins of adult-onset diabetes so we can understand what part lifestyle plays. The evidence needed to clarify the picture is abundant and not difficult to grasp.

First, recall the difference between an inherited disorder and an inherited susceptibility to lifestyle abuse. When a disorder itself is inherited, nothing can be done to prevent the occurrence of that disease. The individual inherits a faulty trait that sooner or later will be expressed. On the other hand, if the only thing inherited is a susceptibility to abuse, then the occurrence of the disease is completely dependent on the occurrence of abuse. If there is no abuse, the disease will never occur. The evidence overwhelmingly supports the classification of adult-onset diabetes as a condition of the latter kind.[10]

Some convincing investigations provide perspective on what kind of lifestyle can lead to the disease. Those studies, carried out in the Middle East, examined Yemenite and Kurdish Jews who had migrated from their homelands to Israel.[11] Among native Yemenites, one case of diabetes was found in every 1,700 people tested. Among native Kurds, no diabetes was detected in 1,000 people examined. When Yemenite immigrants to Israel were examined after twenty-five years of residence, the diabetes rate had increased to one case in every thirty people. The rate among twenty-five-year Kurdish settlers in Israel was one in fifty. Thus in a time period equivalent to just one generation, the average prevalence of diabetes in the two groups of people increased by some fortyfold. There is no way that inheritance could have been responsible for such a dramatic change in such a short time in homogeneous populations. It was a change in environment that caused the increase.

The investigators carried the experiment a bit further and looked into some of the differences between the lifestyle patterns of native Yemenites and those of Yemenite settlers in Israel.[12] Because of the nature of adult-onset diabetes, diet is the lifestyle factor most likely to influence the control mechanisms affected by the disease. When diets were compared between the native Yemenites and the settlers in Israel, the only significant difference found was in the intake of refined sugar: five pounds per person per year in Yemen; fifty-five pounds in Israel. So, a fortyfold increase in the occurrence of diabetes was associated with an elevenfold increase in their intake of sugar.

Even though the results of those studies seem conclusive, it would be good to have some supporting evidence before pinpointing sugar as the prime culprit. Such evidence is readily available. Other studies on the increase in diabetes among primitive peoples who have moved to settings in which their sugar intake is increased have led researchers to draft two "rules" describing the phenomenon.[13] These are:

The Rule of Twenty Years
When people move from areas of dietary deprivation into urban areas where food is freely available, there is a strikingly

constant period of twenty years' exposure to "westernized diets" before diabetes emerges.

The Rule of Ten Per Cent

In those social groups in which diabetes is particularly common, refined sugar typically constitutes more than 10 per cent of total calorie intake in the group.

The sugar intake of the Yemenite settlers, at fifty-five pounds per year, was about eleven per cent of their total calorie intake. The average American today consumes over 20 per cent of his or her total calories as sucrose (common table sugar) plus similar refined sweeteners.[14] (A number of corn derivatives have become popular in recent years as sugar alternatives, primarily in processed foods. Because they are metabolized almost exactly like sucrose, they have to be included with common sugar when assessing its influence on the body's ability to adapt.)

So, if our sugar intake is so much higher than that of the Yemenite settlers, and if sugar intake is the primary cause of diabetes, we might expect that Americans would have a significantly higher incidence of the disease. Indeed, we do. Diabetes now affects over 5 per cent of the American population (more than one in every twenty people) and is still increasing annually in incidence. While this increase has been occurring, have we Americans been increasing our intake of sugar and equivalent sweeteners? Indeed, we have—from about 10 per cent of calories in 1900 to 22 per cent in 1983. In 1875, sugar provided only 5 per cent of calories for the average American.[15]

One other thing we need to know before concluding the case against sugar is whether or not that substance can cause degenerative effects in the body's adaptation system, and whether or not such effects could reasonably be expected to produce diabetes. To do that we have to look a bit more closely at how the body regulates the disposal of sugar from the diet.

When foods containing carbohydrates are consumed and digested, they are assimilated into the circulation and become blood sugar. As that process occurs, the blood-sugar level increases. The increase looks to the body's adaptation mechanisms like an instability, so it reacts to restore the stability it desires— a normal blood-sugar level. The mechanism used to return to stability is release of the hormone insulin into the blood stream. The insulin is able to help dispose of the excess sugar, causing its return to normal levels in the blood. The amount of the hormone released for that purpose depends on how rapidly the concentration of sugar in the blood increases after consumption of dietary carbohydrates. If blood sugar increases very rapidly, the insulin response will be very large. If the blood-sugar increase is slow, the insulin response will be small.

Whatever the amount of insulin release, the purpose of that hormone response is not to fulfill any essential physiological need. In fact, the body never needs more than a very minute amount of the hormone to perform all of its normally required activities. The only purpose for having excess insulin in the blood is to dispose of the excess sugar, to initiate the garbage-collecting process.

What kinds of dietary intake produce rapid blood-sugar increases, and how large can the resulting insulin response be? After eating, blood-sugar levels increase in proportion to the amount of carbohydrate food consumed and the ease with which the carbohydrate components can be digested and assimilated. Simple carbohydrates that require little or no digestion will be quickly assimilated, causing a rapid increase in blood sugar. More complex carbohydrates require considerable digestion before their constituent sugars can be assimilated, so they produce a much slower rise in blood-sugar level. In either case, larger total carbohydrate intakes will give larger blood-sugar responses. Obviously, a large intake of simple sugars (such as regular refined sugar, honey and the several corn derivatives that react like sugar in the body) is most likely to cause rapid blood-sugar responses.

To illustrate, consider that great symbol of American life, apple pie. Cut yourself a generous slice and, as a special treat, add a large scoop of ice cream. If you consume that popular dessert in a typically short time period, the following will occur: its high content of simple refined sugar will send your blood-sugar level shooting up so rapidly that, within thirty minutes, your rate of insulin output will increase one hundredfold.[16]

To put such an increase into perspective, picture the engine of your automobile. It idles at a rate of about 700 revolutions per minute (rpm) when it is running with your foot off the accelerator. That slow idle represents the amount of insulin output required to meet all of your body's normal needs for the hormone. (Remember that insulin amounts over that basal level are needed only to activate garbage collection.) One hundred times the idle speed in your car would be 70,000 rpm. If you could make it run that fast (and if your car would hold together during the experience), that engine speed would take you down the road at a speed of mach 2, or twice the speed of sound.

When you eat that apple pie ala mode, what occurs in your body is roughly equivalent to accelerating your car from idle to a speed of 1,500 miles per hour. Imagine the effect on your car if you were to subject it to such treatment several times a day for twenty years!

One limitation of adaptation mechanisms in the human body is that they are not intended to react continuously to extreme conditions. They cannot maintain internal stability indefinitely if they are continually challenged to the limits of their adaptive capabilities. They are designed to deal with what would be considered, currently and historically, routine changes in the conditions human bodies are exposed to. When the changes become more extreme, the adapative mechanisms can become over-loaded and may malfunction.

Imagine that you live in a third-floor apartment and have a sink with both a leaky faucet and a stopped-up drain. You dispose of the water accumulating in the sink by dipping it out with a pan, running down three flights of stairs and dumping it in the gutter. For you, stability would be a sink that doesn't overflow. You are the mechanism of adaptation. Your living environment adapts to the change (the accumulating water) by your removing some of the water as it collects. If the challenge is not extreme (if the leak is not severe), you can adapt with little difficulty, dipping out a portion now and then and taking it out for disposal. But what if the leak becomes a torrent? Then you will have to spend most of your time running up and down stairs carrying water. There is a limit to how fast you can do that. If the flow continues, you will begin to wear out and, in spite of your most heroic efforts, the sink will finally begin to overflow anyway. Picture yourself on those stairs, taking your last gasping steps before total exhaustion. That is what it's like for your body's adaptation mechanisms when you push them far beyond their intended capabilities.

In simple terms, adult-onset diabetes is the result of a life of what I call insulin abuse: excessive use of the body's insulin control machinery for purposes irrelevant to its essential control responsibilities in the body. That kind of abuse turns a sensitive instrument into a garbage collector. After twenty to forty years (depending on the degree of inherited susceptibility), the machinery wears out for many people and they spend the rest of their lives as diabetics. Of course, not all people who engage in careless dietary practices become diabetics. Like the sturdy silver goblet in my earlier illustration, some people have inherited insulin control systems that can endure a life of abuse without ever malfunctioning. But as the level of abuse and the incidence of diabetes increase in our society, the proportion of such "genetic fortunates" is diminishing.

The only sure way to decrease the risk of becoming a diabetic is to choose a lifestyle that avoids abuse of your body's insulin control system. For many people, that means making a substantial change from their present way of life. It will mean cutting way back on the intake of desserts and other sweets, opting for something other than sugar-sweetened soda pop (or those popular "fruit drinks" and drink mixes that are really almost all sugar), and using fresh instead of canned fruit.

Giving up sugar is a tough decision. In a study of patients who were already diabetic and needed to avoid sugar intake to keep the disease from destroying them, only one out of six was willing to give up sugar. That means that almost 85 per cent refused to abandon the use of sugar even when they knew that they could prolong their lives by doing so. Think how much more difficult that decision is when there is no immediate danger to health and life expectancy.

Why is it so difficult to give up a substance that has no essential nutritional value, yet contributes substantially to disease? How willing are you to eliminate most of the sugar from your life?

Dietary Goals for the United States, adopted by the U.S. Senate in the midseventies, recommended reducing by half the intake of sugar by the American people to a level less than 10 per cent of total calories. That would be about what it was in the year 1900. Are you willing to change your lifestyle that much to be a better steward of your health?

While you're pondering the answer to those questions, I'd like to return to the two conditions discussed earlier and consider their interrelationships with diabetes. Overweight is known to increase significantly the risk of diabetes. In fact one study showed that for every 12 per cent above normal in body weight, the risk of diabetes *doubles*.[17] That cause-and-effect relationship becomes more understandable when we consider the body's insulin responses to high sugar loads. I pointed out that a typical response to such a challenge can increase the rate of insulin output by one hundredfold. In overweight people, the increase is even greater, with three-hundredfold increases common in people who are grossly overweight.[18] Thus, the greater the amount of overweight, the greater the insulin abuse from an equivalent carbohydrate intake—and the more likely that the diet will ultimately lead to destruction of the insulin control system and to diabetes.

There is an obvious association of diabetes as a risk factor in the occurrence of cardiovascular disease, since people with diabetes are significantly more likely to develop CVD than the general population.[19] The two conditions have at least one other aspect in common that may indicate a common origin in the diets of those afflicted. Nondiabetics with heart disease have been shown to exhibit much greater insulin output than normal people subjected to the same challenge of dietary sugar. The degree of hyperinsulism in these patients correlates well with their average level of sugar intake.[20]

At this time, no direct causal relationship has been established. It is known, however, that one of the primary roles of insulin in the control of human metabolism is to direct the conversion of excess calories into fat. We also know that atherosclerosis, a primary symptom in CVD, results from the deposition of fat in the walls of blood vessels. Although more evidence is needed before the relationship can be established conclusively, the emerging picture is one of insulin abuse as a common diet-induced factor in the occurrence of overweight, diabetes and CVD. That possibility, linking three of the most troubling health problems facing our culture, adds to my conviction that choices must be made to minimize insulin abuse.

Lower Bowel Disease

The primary contribution of the diet to the proper functioning of the lower digestive system is a class of indigestible substances collectively termed *fiber*. When such substances are chronically deficient in our diets, a number of different pathological conditions can occur. Without discussing all of these diseases I will illustrate how dietary choices can contribute to another degenerative process.

The human intestine can be visualized as a long tube made of a thin membrane surrounded by a layer of muscle. As digestion occurs, the products of digestion are absorbed through the membrane and are picked up by blood vessels in the muscle layer. To push the digesting food through the intestine, the muscle layer creates a continuous wave of contractions along the length of the tube, a process called peristalsis. Most of the digestion products are absorbed while the food is still in the upper end of the intestine, the small intestine. As peristalsis moves the contents into its lower end, the large intestine, about the only material remaining to be absorbed is water.

The absorption of water is, in fact, a primary role of the large intestine, which is very efficient in doing that. If, however, the contents of the intestine do not include some kind of material that will hold water and prevent its complete absorption, they will quickly become dehydrated and very solid, a condition commonly known as constipation. The mechanism of peristalsis is designed to transport semisolid contents, not hard lumps. When constipation occurs, the muscular effort required to move the solid contents is considerably greater, putting substantial strain on the intestinal wall. If such excessive strain is allowed to persist as a way of life for many years, the muscle wall can weaken and finally gave way, allowing an outpouching of the inner membrane. Such outpouches are called diverticula (plural), and the condition when they occur is called diverticulosis. Diverticula often remain essentially unnoticed, causing severe symptoms only when they become infected. Such infection, called diverticulitis, is a frequent consequence of diverticulosis and can be extremely painful. It can be accompanied by a number of potentially serious consequences.

From a number of different lines of evidence, the primary factor contributing to the cause of diverticular disease seems to be a deficiency of fiber in the diet. Dietary fiber has unique properties for promoting water retention in the lower bowel and preventing constipation and diverticulosis.

Fiber intake in Western society since the turn of this century has decreased as a result of an increase in our lifestyle options. In 1900 most calories consumed in this country came from foods containing high contents of dietary fiber, particularly unrefined cereal grains and certain vegetables. Today the two main sources of calories in the average American diet are fat and sugar, between them contributing almost two-thirds of total calorie intake. Neither source contributes *any* dietary fiber.

Eighty years ago, we had no alternative but to eat high-fiber diets. Little else was available. Today we have a multitude of choices—and we're making a lot of wrong ones.

As a consequence, diverticular disease is the most common disease of the large intestine. In Western cultures, it is now reported to affect one in every ten people over the age of forty and one in three over the age of sixty. Before this century, the disease was rare even in developed countries. Today, in Third World societies, it remains rare.[21]

Lower bowel disease continues to increase as we continue to opt for the good life. To prevent the degenerative effects that lead to diverticulosis, overweight, diabetes and cardiovascular disease, we need a radical shift in what we shall eat and what we shall drink. That is the topic of the next chapter.

5 Eating to Stay Well

*T*HIS CHAPTER IS ABOUT THE PREVENTION *OF POTENTIAL DISEASE,* not the treatment of existing disease. Anyone with some condition requiring diet therapy should seek the counsel of a qualified physician. Although I will be discussing weight-loss dieting as an aspect of prevention, the management of true obesity is a medical problem that should be attempted only under the supervision of a medical professional.

To establish the logic for preventive diets, we should first review the bodily needs that must be satisfied from the foods we eat. Quite apart from satisfying whatever cravings and tastes we may have cultivated, what are we trying to accomplish when we eat? We have three essential requirements—energy, tissue replacement or repair, and metabolic regulation. (We have already discussed a fourth requirement, fiber, which only affects the digestive system.) Most food is used to provide energy for the body's metabolic functions. Much of the rest, primarily protein and some minerals, is dedicated to the construction of tissues. What remains, a minute fraction of the total, maintains the body's supply of essential regulators, mainly the vitamins and a number of minerals.

As I mentioned in the preceding chapter, a disproportionate amount of concern in our society is dedicated to vitamins. The same could be said generally of protein. We have been led to believe that protein deficiencies in our diets constitute a primary risk to health. Yet protein malnutrition is virtually unheard of in this country. From the diets I have analyzed, only two nutritional deficiencies (except for fiber, already discussed) occur in Americans with any regularity. They are both minerals: *iron* (mostly in women of childbearing age) and *calcium* (mostly in adults who have abandoned the use of milk). Both can be corrected by adjusting the diet or by taking mineral supplements. Thus I see little value in considering vitamins, minerals or protein in any detail in a discussion of diet as a factor in disease prevention today.[1] Where then do our problems lie?

Dietary choices that lead to degenerative disease almost always involve foods that provide energy. Yet in designing alternatives to those destructive choices, we must bear in mind that the body's demand for energy is not going to disappear just because we decide to play around with its sources of fuel. Whatever we do, our first priority will be to supply the right fuel to the right places in the right amounts at the right time. No matter what other goals we might have (elimination of excess body fat, for example), those goals cannot interfere with this priority for fuel.

One other fact should be clear. We do not have a whole series of different dietary patterns, each leading to a different disease. We have a single diet, generally characteristic of our times and broadly destructive in its influence. Prevention thus means identifying its destructive elements and designing an alternative that meets all of the body's fundamental needs. Such a diet will be different from the one that characterizes the good life. It will unquestionably require hard choices.

Earlier I defined three major priorities in dietary choices of the good life: taste, convenience and appearance. These priorities become quick casualties in a prevention diet. Why do we drink soda pop instead of water when we're thirsty? Why do we eat butter and salt on popcorn? Simply because we prefer the taste. Why are fast-food outlets so popular? Why are canned foods so abundant when modern transportation and refrigeration make fresh foods almost universally available? Primarily because they are convenient. Anyone who has ever heard a chorus of "Yech" or "Ugh" as food was placed on the table knows that appearance is very important. Although a prevention diet need not be unappetizing in taste or appearance, nor a drag on our busy schedules, we must recognize that the priorities of the good life must be confronted if we want to stay well.

Dietary advice typically comes in one of two forms. The most common form provides what I call "eating instructions," detailed regimens outlining what to eat, how much and when. Such instructions are what you get in the multitude of books, articles and sundry other sources of advice on how to lose weight. A former captive of a diet that produced undesirable results (overweight, diabetes or whatever), the dieter now becomes captive to eating instructions. The choices aren't really his or hers, but those of the adviser.

The other form of dietary advice is what I call diet logic, a foundation of fundamental principles on which a person can build a sensible program of dietary choices. This is the approach I use when giving dietary advice and, in my opinion, it is the only approach that promotes responsible health management. So, this book will not provide any diets. Instead I want to teach you how to make your own sensible choices. It is your life, not mine. The decisions that will help to sustain that life should also be yours, not mine.

Although the general principles of prevention dieting are the same whatever an individual's health goals, weight-loss dieting does have some unique requirements. So I will consider prevention dieting in two segments, one dealing with weight loss, the other with prevention in general.

Weight-loss Dieting

I believe a "diet" is, for most people, a secondary factor in weight management. The primary factor is the willingness of individuals to identify, confront and conquer the obstacles that stand between them and permanent weight loss. Those obstacles are almost always emotional rather than physiological in character. In my experience, if a person is not committed to dealing with those obstacles first, the diet becomes of little consequence.

Without question, the biggest single cause of failure in losing weight is lack of commitment. The same is true of other failures to change lifestyle. The challenge to me in helping people manage their lifestyles is to provide convincing strategies for promoting commitment. Because those strategies are common to all the aspects of health management that we will be considering, I prefer to pursue the matter of commitment separately, after discussing the physical causes and effects. In the final chapter I will provide a biblical foundation for maintaining commitment to the stewardship of health. It will supplement my other arguments and strategies for making lifestyle change the means of preserving health. Given one's commitment to that process, though, an understanding of the principles can make the process considerably easier to implement.

Physiologically, the goal of weight-loss dieting is to provide the minimum requirements of the body for continued normal function, while sustaining a deficit in total calorie intake. The deficit will then be made up from stores of body fat, resulting in safe and effective weight loss. What are the minimum requirements of the body for normal function? What is an appropriate calorie deficit? That is, how much can you reduce your total calorie intake and still meet all of those requirements?

These questions don't have simple answers. Minimum requirements and allowable deficits vary from person to person. Although they can be estimated on an individual basis using personal characteristics and standard formulas, that's not really necessary for our purposes here. All we need are some general principles for making lifestyle changes that will promote the loss of weight.

These principles are simple to develop and to understand. Average Americans today consume about 43 per cent of their total calories as fat and another 22 per cent as sugar (or other similar sweeteners).[2] Thus, almost two-thirds of the average diet in this country is provided by two substances that are basically nothing but second-rate fuel sources. Further, too much of them can contribute significantly to body fat.

If you were the diet consultant, what kind of logic would you propose to lose weight? Consider first what you want to accomplish: elimination of calories that have no value either for meeting the continuous fuel demand of the brain or for supplying other nutritional requirements. In the current American diet, the majority of the fat and sugar qualify for elimination under those conditions. Except for a few grams per day (a total of fifty to one hundred calories), fat is completely nonessential. And, as we discovered in our earlier discussions, the way sugar is consumed in our society today, the resulting insulin responses divert much of that potentially useful brain fuel into the garbage heap.

Of course, no one needs to eliminate that great a proportion of total calorie intake in order to accomplish desirable weight loss. For the average person, reducing calories by 20 per cent would result in losing about one pound per week, an excellent target for most people. The point is that there are plenty of useless calories in the typical diet to choose from in establishing a deficit. In fact, the more of those useless calories you can eliminate over and above the amount desired for losing weight, the more opportunity you will have to substitute foods that will help make your weight-loss diet into an effective prevention diet.

For example, elimination of 35 grams of sugar (seven teaspoons, or the amount in one twelve-ounce serving of regular soda pop) will yield, without substitution, a 140-calorie deficit. Or, if you wanted to substitute two slices of whole-grain bread for the same amount of sugar, the calorie intake would be the same, but it would include 24 grams of an ideal (complex) form of carbohydrate for fuel, a significant contribution of protein, vitamins and minerals, plus about 15 per cent of your total recommended intake of dietary fiber. Elimination of three teaspoons of butter, margarine or other fat will yield a deficit of 100 calories, without substitution. If you substitute two cups of broccoli for the same amount of fat, you can obtain (at no increase in calories) 17 grams of excellent carbohydrate fuel, 11 grams of protein, three times the Recommended Dietary Allowance (RDA) of vitamin C, twice the RDA of vitamin A, half the recommended minimum daily intake of potassium, one-fourth the RDA of calcium, phosphorus and iron (only 15 per cent of the iron for women, who need more), plus significant contributions of other vitamins, minerals and fiber.

In general, major sources of sugar in the typical diet tend to be obvious and easily identified. For example, it is estimated that over one-third of all sugar now consumed in this country is in soft drinks. Fat sources, on the other hand, tend to be more obscure. Yet some of our favorite sources of sugar are also large contributors of fat. For example, a one-ounce chocolate bar contains over two teaspoons (90 calories) of fat. One cup of high-quality commercial ice cream contains about two tablespoons (215 calories) of fat. An average piece of pecan pie contains about the same amount. Many other desserts and sweets contain substantial amounts of fat. So the simplest way to begin removing useless calories from the diet is to eliminate, or greatly reduce, the obvious sources of sugar. Many people will discover that the simple strategy of eliminating high-sugar items from the diet will be sufficient for losing weight without any other significant change in eating patterns.

Fat is a more subtle dietary constituent than sugar, both in its high-calorie density (calories per unit volume) and in its tendency to remain unnoticed when it is present but to be greatly missed in its absence. Fat adds significantly to the palatability of foods, without being obvious. The best cuts of beef, for example, are generously "marbled" with streaks of fat in the meat. As a result, a choice cut of prime rib will have over 80 per cent of its total calories contributed by its fat content. Meats, in fact, are major contributors of fat for most North Americans today. Eighty per cent of the calories in frankfurters come from fat, 84 per cent in pork sausage, 79 per cent in bacon, and about 72 per cent in hamburger.[3]

So another strategy for eliminating significant amounts of useless calories from the diet is to cut back on meat intake. If you undertake a substantial reduction, however, several precautions should be observed. For many people, meat is the major source of protein. Although most of us consume far more protein than we need, care should be taken to assure that protein content remains adequate if a major portion of meat is to be eliminated. Alternative sources of good protein that are low in fat are poultry (skinned), fish and dairy products derived from skim milk.

The other precaution to be noted in the elimination of meat from the diet is that red meats presently provide the majority of the iron for most North Americans. The complete elimination of this source can present a problem for women, who have a high requirement for that mineral during their child-bearing years. My usual recommendation is that dieters select their major sources of iron from among the following—lean red meat (trimmed of all fat), beans or dark green vegetables (broccoli, spinach, etc.)—and then adjust their protein intake as necessary. I recommend supplemental iron if the diet is not certain to provide adequately for the need.

Other sources of fat that could reasonably be eliminated will be more difficult to identify. Certainly, frying or deep-frying foods adds significantly to their fat content. Salad dressings, dips, sauces and gravies are typically high in fats. Nuts and seeds are very high in fat. Regular cheeses and other dairy products not made with skim milk also have a high fat content. Many commercially prepared foods contain a lot more fat than we realize. You will find it useful to read labels carefully when you are shopping for such items. And, of course, restaurants and fast-food outlets are veritable bonanzas of dietary fat. A trip through the golden arches for a Big Mac and regular fries will net you 44.5 grams of dietary fat (more than three tablespoons—400 calories).[4]

The logic of weight-loss dieting is, thus, remarkably simple. People in this country are overweight mainly because of their excessive intake of useless calories, primarily in the form of sugar and fat. They can begin to burn up the body fat that useless calories produce by eliminating these calorie sources in the diet. Substituting more healthy foods (fruits, vegetables, whole-grain cereal products, low-fat dairy products) for some of those useless calories and maintaining a modest deficit in total calorie intake (perhaps 500 calories per day, which will give about one pound per week in *fat* loss) will provide a good basis for healthy weight loss.

A few other strategies will help make this kind of diet easier to implement. First, to reiterate an important point made earlier, in dieting it is essential that energy levels in the body be kept high enough to meet all of its needs. "Loss of energy" is probably the most frequent reason that people terminate their diets. For the purpose of maintaining one's energy, the best fuel by far is carbohydrate. So the only sensible approach requires that reducing diets be *high* in carbohydrates, a strategy that contradicts much popular opinion, which disdains carbohydrate as "fattening." That opinion has no basis in scientific fact. It is, in fact, a significant contributor to the high failure rate in weight management in this country today.

Carbohydrate is the body's best source of fuel. When you limit carbohydrate in your diet, you substantially restrict this energy resource (frequently promoting fatigue) and often compel the body to burn up its own tissues to meet the energy demand. I have polled groups of weight-conscious people for those who have purchased a hamburger sandwich, discarded the bun and eaten the meat. The proportion who admit to this practice is very high. They are almost always shocked to learn that they have discarded a 100-calorie bun, which they *think* will help make them overweight, in favor of eating a 300-calorie hamburger patty (215 calories of which come from fat) which*will* help make them overweight. In the bun, they have thrown away about 20 grams of good carbohydrate fuel.

The fact is, not all carbohydrates are a problem for weight-loss dieters—only those that provoke excessive insulin responses (sugar and similar sweeteners). Carbohydrates that are more moderate in their influence on insulin control machinery (such as the more complex carbohydrates found in grain products and most vegetables) serve a critical role as sources of essential fuel to help the dieter maintain energy levels. These carbohydrates should be emphasized in *any* diet in which the maintenance of energy levels is important. In fact, I recommend the same kind of high-carbohydrate diets (with appropriate adjustments in total calories) both for weight-loss dieters and for long-distance runners. Both need to maintain energy at high levels in the face of unique physiological demands.

By my definition, "high carbohydrate" means that 60 per cent or more of the calories in the diet come from carbohydrates. To achieve that percentage, such foods as cereal products, fruits and vegetables should predominate.

One additional strategy can be employed to help stabilize energy availability during the day and minimize the adaptation responses that provoke hunger. That strategy requires that you distribute your food intake into five or six meals or snacks each day. I will have more to say about that strategy in the following section.

Finally, I want to comment about cost as it relates to dieting. I am aware that dieting can become an expensive project for some people. What most people don't stop to consider is that the high cost is typically not a matter of necessity but of convenience. When you buy special "dietary" foods, you are paying for the convenience of not having to make your own decisions about the content of the foods you eat. Or you are paying to avoid, as much as possible, having to give up the good life. Low-calorie diets, if well designed, can be low-cost diets. After all, such a diet needs to minimize some of the most expensive foods (meat, cheese and snack items) and maximize some of the least expensive (cereal grains and vegetables).

To help you with the selection of foods to be included in your diet, I have compiled nutritional data from several hundred common food items into a list of fifty-nine food groups. These food groups are listed in the appendix, with information on their calorie content, the distribution of their calories in protein, carbohydrate and fat, and some comments about their overall contribution to nutrition.

Prevention Dieting

Because both overweight and degenerative disease are common results of the typical Western diet, much of what was said about a weight-loss diet also applies to prevention diets. Primarily, they should minimize useless calories, sugar and other refined carbohydrates that promote insulin abuse, and fat. Foods substituted for the sugar and fat should be high in complex carbohydrates and should contain some good sources of dietary fiber. For most of us, to minimize the risk of hypertension, sodium (salt) intake should be reduced to about one-third of its present intake. Contrary to popular belief, the changes required to accomplish those goals need not be drastic. First, to eat healthfully we do not have to do our shopping in health-food stores. The supermarkets (from which we buy many of the things that are killing us) sell everything we need to stay healthy. It's a matter of making the right choices. In addition, healthy eating does not have to be a drag. For many people it will be different and sometimes necessarily less convenient. But good, nutritious food can be prepared to make it both appealing and tasty. In a word, abandoning the dietary good life does not mean that life has to become less pleasant.

Unquestionably, for most people, the most important aspect of prevention dieting will be not what is included in the diet but what is eliminated. From what we have seen about how our diets contribute to major degenerative disease, it should be evident that a reduction in the intake of sugar and other refined carbohydrates is the number one priority.

The most effective strategy for accomplishing this goal requires attention not just to what and how much you eat, but to when you eat it. Several times I have mentioned the brain's need for a constant supply of fuel, in the form of blood sugar. Whenever that supply comes up short, one of the body's adaptation mechanisms, the stress response, reacts to correct the situation.

One such stress mechanism is the "crave" reaction, a stimulus intended to motivate feeding behavior. That stimulus is a major factor in motivating people to snack on sweets. There can also be purely emotional components to such cravings, which I will discuss later in the discussion of commitment.

Dietary choices can help suppress the physiological component of the crave response in two major ways. First, a prime cause of temporary blood-sugar deficit is an insulin-mediated overreaction in response to large intakes of sugar. The large output of insulin provoked by such sugar burdens sometimes removes the excess blood sugar too effectively and causes a temporary shortage. So sugar intake itself can be a major cause of a subsequent craving for sugar. If those cravings are satisfied by another large intake of sugar, the process can start again. It becomes a feast-famine cycle throughout the day, characterized by repeated episodes of stress as the body adapts each time to a deficit in the brain's fuel supply. Obviously, this source of craving can be eliminated by avoiding the intake of sugar in large doses.

A second way to suppress the craving for sugar is to prevent an excessive drain on the blood-sugar supply as it is being used for its intended purpose, as fuel for the body's critical functions. In an average person, the brain uses more than three and a half grams of blood sugar per hour to meet its constant energy demand and that of other tissues in the body which compete for that blood-sugar supply. At normal levels, the total average blood volume can hold only about five grams of sugar. So, without fairly regular supplements from the diet, this fuel supply can become depleted in a short time. The result will be a stress response, including craving, as the body reacts to make a correction.

The strategy for eliminating craving has two elements. First, when we consume carbohydrates (which should constitute the majority of the calories in the diet), those carbohydrates should be complex and unrefined. That way they will tend to promote slower and more extended blood-sugar responses after eating. Second, if we eat more frequently, the diet will be able to provide a more continuous supply of blood sugar and will greatly diminish the possibility of between-meal cravings. I recommend, as in weight-loss dieting, a general practice of diverting some calories from meals to between-meal snacks. The foods used in such snacks, like the meals, should promote sustained blood-sugar responses.

The excessive amount of sodium consumed in the typical modern diet is due primarily to an acquired taste that has become conditioned to misinterpret the real needs of the body for the substance. In this case, as in so many others we have discussed, an important mechanism for adaptation has been abused until it malfunctions. Scientific studies have shown that the level of salt intake in humans is reflected in its excretion in the saliva.[5] This mechanism provides a "salt background" against which the taste of the foods you eat will be compared. When the amount of salt in the diet is low, excretion in the saliva is reduced and the foods you eat will taste saltier. On the other hand, if your intake of salt is high, excretion in the saliva will be greater and much more salt will be needed on your food for you to be able to taste it.

Where did we acquire our "need" for high levels of salt? First, when our taste level was initially acquired, most of us were in no position to do anything about it. We were infants, essentially force-fed with whatever our parents (and the baby-food industry) decided was good for us. Now the food-processing industry sustains an elevated salt level in the foods they manufacture—both to satisfy the exaggerated taste levels of the majority of Americans and sometimes as an expedient in the manufacturing process.

The strategy for reducing salt intake is simple. All you have to do is begin to cut back systematically on your salt intake. You won't even have to sacrifice your enjoyment of the taste; the taste-discrimination mechanism will adjust in a few weeks to give you the same sense of flavor with less salt. In addition to avoiding the saltshaker, I recommend that certain major offenders be dealt with first: canned foods, particularly vegetables, soups and entrees (many of which have 1,000 to 1,500 milligrams of sodium per serving); fast-food sandwiches (some of which contain over 1,500 milligrams of sodium, an amount considered a desirable *maximum* per day to minimize the risk of hypertension); salted snack items such as potato chips and corn chips; many sauces and seasonings; and salted meats. This list is by no means exhaustive, but it probably includes most of the categories that provide the bulk of salt consumed in our society today. The labels on commercially prepared foods often give information on sodium content.

Without doubt, the most universal deficiency in the Western diet today is fiber. The best single source of dietary fiber available in the food supply is bran, the material that makes up the surface layer of the seeds of grains such as wheat and rice. When those grains are refined, the surface layer is removed and, with it, 70 to 85 per cent of the fiber. There is no fiber at all in fats, meats or dairy products—and none in sugar. Most of the calories we consume thus come without *any* associated fiber.

The only way to correct that deficiency is to eat foods that are significant contributors of fiber. These include (besides whole grains and their products) peas and beans, nuts and certain fruits (particularly berries, dried fruits, bananas and pears). All of these foods are readily available in your local supermarket. Any of them would make excellent substitutes for the useless calories that currently dominate the typical diet. My only caution would be that because nuts have a high fat content, the fiber in them may not be worth the additional calories they contribute.

What about protein, vitamins and minerals? Aren't they also important? Of course. But if you make the adjustments I have recommended, most often the resulting diet will be adequate in all essential nutrients. Unless it is very low in total calories, your diet will probably not require any further supplementation.

6 Alcohol, Tobacco, Caffeine

*I*N ONE OF MY SEMINARS A FEW YEARS AGO THERE WAS A YOUNG woman in her late teens who had been a regular user of popular street drugs. By the time I met her, she had abandoned the use of those drugs and had sought a physician's help in dealing with a problem of chronic stress. She was referred to me for counseling in lifestyle management. During one of the sessions, we concentrated on her current intake of caffeine. When she became aware of her high daily intake of that substance (over 1,000 milligrams) and of the drug's powerful stimulant action, she exclaimed, "My gosh! I'm still a hophead."

Substance abuse is rampant in our society. The main body of abusers are solid citizens, like you and me, who would probably bristle at being given such a label. I define a *substance* as any exogenous chemical (one introduced from outside the body) that alters the normal progress of human metabolism, that is, the chemical processes of life. Of course, the number of such chemicals employed for this purpose in our society is extremely large. Most of them are medicinal drugs used in the practice of medicine. Some are illegal drugs. Some are legal nonprescription drugs used by a large proportion of North Americans on a regular basis. I will restrict my discussion to three substances from this last category because of their widespread use and abuse, and because of their potential for promoting degenerative disease. These three substances are alcohol, tobacco (specifically from cigarettes) and caffeine.

The consequences of substance abuse go far beyond the promotion of degenerative disease. I want to confine my discussion primarily to the direct or indirect participation of the above three substances in the degeneration of the body's in-born tendency to be healthy. To do that, it will be necessary to establish a perspective on use and abuse that goes beyond the usual definitions. I hope that such a perspective will give some food for thought to many people who consider themselves to be safely casual users.

As a foundation, I would like to emphasize that there is no neatly defined point at which use becomes abuse. Substance abuse is typically evaluated in terms of gross physical, emotional or social ends. It would be foolish, however, to believe that the overt symptoms of degenerative disease are only the initial stages of a disease process. Quite the contrary. Those states are almost always the result of long-term progressive degeneration. So, for every person who is identified as a victim of substance abuse, from overt symptoms, there are multitudes of others with more subtle signs who have probably suffered some degenerative effects.

How shall we define the term *abuse*? Substance abuse usually conjures up the image of some kid in an abandoned building, with a candle and blackened spoon, intent on his daily ritual of shooting heroin. But abuse can actually come in innocent-looking disguises. Insulin abuse, as seen earlier, can occur in the simple act of eating a piece of pie. Why was it *abuse*? Because the body's adaptation mechanisms were forced to function beyond the limits that normal environmental variations would require. What were the consequences? Exhaustion of the body's ability to adapt or a malfunctioning of normal metabolism, both of them degenerative processes that lead to disease. As far as possible, I will continue to use this same general definition.

Alcohol

Alcohol is a drug. The fact that it is distributed widely and consumed legally in the adult population; the fact that it is in common use, with almost three gallons of pure alcohol (the equivalent of six gallons of liquor, twenty gallons of wine or seventy gallons of beer) being consumed per person per year in the United States; the fact that it is widely accepted as a routine part of our lives—none of that alters one simple fundamental of chemistry and physiology: alcohol is a drug. Two-thirds of the adult population and three-fourths of high-school students admit to some use of it.

Alcohol is also a widely abused drug. Fifteen per cent of all adult drinkers (10 per cent of the total adult population) meet the minimum criteria for having a drinking problem. Of even greater concern is the fact that, by the criteria set for them, *more than* 10 per cent of *all* tenth to twelfth graders can be considered problem drinkers.[1]

The social consequences of alcohol abuse are enormous. But our concern here is with the biological consequences and its influence on health. To assess that influence, let's start with how our bodies deal with alcohol and what effects it can impose on the adaptation mechanisms that preserve health.

Like most of what we ingest, alcohol is absorbed into the blood by the digestive system. During its stay in the body, it exhibits its most familiar effect—the depression of certain brain functions. That effect, called cerebral depression, is what drinkers typically experience, depending on blood-alcohol levels, as the various stages of inebriation. Alcohol remains in the body until it can be eliminated by the process of detoxification.

The purpose of detoxification, an adaptation mechanism, is to rid the body of any potentially toxic substances to which it is exposed. As with all adaptation mechanisms, detoxification equips the body to deal with *reasonable* environmental exposures to toxic substances. It can be overloaded if the exposures are excessive. As seen earlier, the two primary consequences of such overloads are failure to adapt to the total exposure and degeneration of the adaptation system itself, resulting in a permanent disability of the system. Either of those consequences can increase the chances of degenerative disease.

The most familiar disease from alcohol abuse is cirrhosis of the liver, a degenerative condition characterized by destruction of liver tissue and loss of liver function. The occurrence and the severity of this disease are in direct proportion to the level of abuse. The extent of abuse also seems to parallel the total level of alcohol consumption in the society. For example, in the thirty-six years following the repeal of prohibition in 1932, per capita alcohol consumption among people over age fifteen in the United States increased by 150 per cent. In the same period, deaths from cirrhosis increased by more than 100 per cent.[2]

The primary effect of alcohol abuse occurs in the liver because the liver is the body's primary organ of detoxification. Any time a chemical substance must be detoxified in the body, the liver typically deals with the substance in one of two ways: (1) conversion of the substance to a harmless by-product that can be excreted through the kidneys and eliminated in the urine; or (2) conversion of the substance to a form that can fit in with the body's normal metabolism. Alcohol detoxification is of this second type.

When this occurs, the usual end product is a fuel substance which (depending on the body's need for energy at the time) can be used to generate energy or can be stored away, typically as fat. This is accomplished with relative ease when the blood levels of alcohol are moderate. In the first step of detoxification, the process generates very briefly a toxic compound called acetaldehyde. Because conversion proceeds so rapidly at low blood-alcohol levels, this toxic material never accumulates in high enough concentrations to have any detrimental effect. As the level of alcohol in the body increases, however, the metabolic resources necessary for the conversion of acetaldehyde become overwhelmed, and this toxic substance begins to accumulate. As it accumulates, the detoxification process slows down, so the alcohol concentration in the blood remains high for longer periods. In addition, during such metabolic overload, the end product of detoxification is almost exclusively fat.

For the average drinker, the only *noticeable* effect of alcohol excess is what is commonly known as a hangover, an unpleasant but temporary consequence of alcohol toxicity and catabolism (breakdown in the liver). But not all of the effects of alcohol toxicity are temporary, nor are they restricted to that one out of every ten Americans over age fifteen classified as a problem drinker. Often our ability to detect degenerative effects is sufficiently unrefined that such effects do not become noticeable until they have progressed to the point of significant damage.

Alcohol is a very powerful and toxic chemical. Even a level of intake considered moderate by social standards can be abusive as far as the body's adaptation mechanisms are concerned. A common misconception, for example, is the idea that liver damage, leading to cirrhosis in the extreme, is the only serious health consequence of alcohol abuse. Alcohol can cause a multitude of different degenerative effects.

In the past, most of these effects were studied in detail only

among alcoholics and were considered to be specific consequences of alcoholism. As research methods improve, however,
it is being shown that some effects represent a continuum of
degenerative damage—with small but distinguishable effects
observed at lower alcohol intakes, progressing to severe symptoms at very high intakes.

Evidence shows, for example, that the use of alcohol can cause
damage to the cardiovascular system. This is seen primarily in
three disease conditions: hypertension (high blood pressure),
stroke and alcoholic cardiomyopathy, a nonspecific degeneration
of heart structure and function with no other detectable cause
than alcohol intake. Another common manifestation of cardiovascular disease, atherosclerosis, appears to occur *less* frequently
in moderate drinkers than in abstainers. The possible cause of
this effect is still a matter of speculation. Because of other dele-
terious effects of alcohol intake on the cardiovascular system and
other systems in the body, however, no one is prepared at this
time to justify alcohol intake on the basis of that observation.

Alcohol has also been shown to injure the endocrine system,
the system that produces and uses hormones. For example, in
males alcohol reduces the level of the hormone testosterone, the
mediator of male sexual function. This is known to result in sexual impotence, loss of libido and progressive "feminization," the
degeneration of male sexual characteristics and development of
female characteristics.

Alcohol can also damage the nervous system. Investigations
have demonstrated the occurrence of defects in the brains of
alcoholics and of heavy social drinkers. Such defects include
changes in brain architecture, decreases in blood flow and ab-
normalities in brain-wave activity as recorded in electroencepha-
lograms. In addition, neuropsychological functioning—that is,
the ability to recognize, associate and remember things—has
been found to be diminished in regular alcohol drinkers. The

loss of function appears to be well correlated with the level of alcohol use, *with some impairment observable in moderate social drinkers* and an increasing level of impairment observed with increases in average alcohol intake.

The evidence for neuropsychological damage from alcohol is significant for two reasons. First, it is an example of what is almost certainly true about alcohol's general effect on the body. That is, the damage alcohol causes is directly related to the individual's average level of consumption. We do not see a direct expression of most negative effects in the more moderate drinkers simply because we have no sufficiently sensitive tests for the defects at that level. But at least in the brain, we know that physical defects occur in moderate social drinkers because we can detect the loss of intellectual function. It would be most surprising if the nervous system were the only system in the human body that was harmed at moderate levels of intake.

Second, the neuropsychological evidence is significant because moderate and heavier drinkers in the United States today comprise one-third of the entire adult population of the country *(and almost 50 per cent of all high-school students).* So we're not talking about something that affects some small segment of the American people. We're talking about a major national condition. This means that one-third of the people at the controls of social, economic and political life in this country are losing some cognitive function because of their alcohol intake. Half of the young people who may be assuming that control in the future have already lost some cognitive capacity because of their use of alcohol.

To be so popular in the face of the overwhelming evidence of its destructive effects (and I haven't even mentioned more than ten million full-blown alcoholics) alcohol must have a tremendous appeal. What is it? It has no value at all for health and nutrition. It cannot be considered harmless even in moderation. Its obvious appeal is pleasure—or, as is more often the case, the elimination of unpleasantness. This stems from alcohol's primary drug property, cerebral depression, which helps a drinker to "relax" or, in more correct terms, to escape reality. I will have more to say about that in a later chapter on stress.

One could probably achieve a unanimous consensus on the proposition that to seek pleasure is not wrong if, in the seeking, no harm is done. How could that consensus be applied in the matter of alcohol use? Applying a cost/benefit approach, perhaps we could convince ourselves that a little bit of brain degeneration is acceptable if the pleasure is great enough. Or perhaps we would allow a slightly higher risk of hypertension if escape from reality is deemed absolutely necessary. Such rationalizations, however, do not change facts. The pleasure and the escape are always temporary. The physical degeneration is frequently permanent. Whether you drink and how much you drink are matters of personal choice. You should know that your choices in these matters have the potential for serious consequences.

Finally, I hope you are as shocked and dismayed as I was when I learned how many teen-agers are heavy drinkers. Where do young people get the idea that drinking alcohol is acceptable? It is a social norm in our society, a norm set by an adult population that thinks it is acceptable for *them* to drink but not acceptable for kids. Is that a valid distinction? Even if it were, are teen-agers emotionally advanced enough to accept it?

Let's not fool ourselves. Three-fourths of all high-school students drink *because two-thirds of all adults drink*. We can bemoan the teen-age drinking problem, pour money into studying it, have meetings on it and write articles about it. But it will begin to go away only when the adults change their attitude toward drinking. Teen-agers model their choices about alcohol after the choices adults make—only teen-age choices are made with considerably less capacity for mature judgment.

Tobacco

When I give a lecture that includes a discussion of the health risks of cigarette smoking (the only use of tobacco in our society that puts a major segment of the population at risk), I ask a smoker in the audience to read these words from the cigarette package: "Warning: The Surgeon General has determined that cigarette smoking is dangerous to your health." Then I ask, "Do you believe that?" Perhaps surprisingly, the answer I almost always get is yes.

When asked why, if they believe it, they continue to smoke, most often the answer is "Because I don't think it will happen to me."

Essentially, cigarette smokers are a group of high-stakes gamblers, betting they can beat the odds. Every year, hundreds of thousands of them lose the bet. Over 100 thousand of them this year will get lung cancer and, within five years, 90 per cent of those victims will be dead.[3] Many other losers will have heart attacks, strokes or other forms of cardiovascular malfunction. Some of them will get emphysema, a disabling, progressively degenerative disease of the lungs, which causes the individual to suffocate slowly.

Cigarette smoking is so well established as a health risk that there is little I can present that is not already common knowledge. It is by far the most frequent cause of lung disease among Americans, particularly lung cancer, which is now increasing faster than any other disease in our culture. Smokers are almost ten times more likely to get the disease than nonsmokers. Smoking is a major factor that increases the chance for cardiovascular disease, with smokers at roughly twice the risk of nonsmokers.[4] Yet all of that information is well known in our society and accepted as fact even by most smokers themselves. Why in the world do they continue smoking? To answer that question, let's look at the physiology of addiction.

When we were considering alcohol abuse, I dealt only minimally with the problem of alcohol addiction, even though there are more people addicted to alcohol than any other drug. Unquestionably, addiction is the most severe form of alcohol abuse, constituting a tremendous social and economic problem. Yet alcohol addiction is only the ultimate state in a continuum from light intake to extreme abuse. Addicts constitute a small percentage of all users. With alcohol, it is the process, not its terminal consequence, that needs to receive our attention when considering how to preserve health.

On the other hand, we must regard virtually *all* regular cigarette smokers as addicts. Whatever their level of use, they are addicted to the substance. With cigarettes, it's not a matter of moderation as opposed to abuse. Use *is* abuse in cigarette smoking. While light smokers have a lower risk of disease than heavy smokers, even light smokers have a significantly higher risk of disease than nonsmokers. Light smokers remain smokers for the same reason that heavy smokers remain smokers: addiction. Thus, although it is possible for most people to prevent the risk of alcohol addiction by exercising moderation in their drinking, the only way to prevent addiction in the use of cigarettes is abstinence. You're either a nonsmoker or you're an addict.[5]

Many people have a poor understanding of what it means to be addicted to a substance and of how *addiction* differs from *habituation* and *dependence*.[6] For the purposes of this discussion, let me give the following definitions.

Habituation: Need for continued use of a substance in which the need is of predominantly emotional origin.

Dependence: Need for continued use of a substance in which the need has its basis in a *substance-induced* alteration in the body's physiological mechanisms of adaptation.

Addiction: Dependence as defined above, with two important distinctions: (1) withdrawal of the substance is associated with severely unpleasant symptoms; and (2) the addict is aware that a return to substance use will eliminate those symptoms.

It is now generally accepted that cigarette smoking, as it is commonly practiced in our society, is an addiction. Classification of smokers as addicts provides a much better understanding of why they persist in the practice when the evidence of its health risks is so overwhelming.

While the physical origins of cigarette addiction are strong, the emotional component is also important. Most of us have observed people whose smoking patterns are directly related to their level of tension. In fact, the elevated health risk (especially the risk for CVD) in heavy smokers may be due as much to their stress as to their smoking per se.

Preventing the harmful consequences of cigarette smoking is reducible to a formula: If you are a nonsmoker, don't start; if you are a smoker, quit. Of course, while the formula is simple, its implementation is anything but easy. Anyone who has quit smoking knows the difficulty. But too many hard-core smokers have quit successfully for anyone to believe that this addiction cannot be overcome by anyone who really wants to fight it. There is no such thing as a person who *can't* quit smoking—only people who *won't*.

Why won't they? Inevitably we come back to the matter of pleasure, or the avoidance of unpleasantness. Consider the unpleasantness experienced in withdrawal from cigarette smoking. Is it a sign that something unhealthy is happening in the body? Not at all. Quite the contrary. It is a sign that the body is attempting to reestablish its natural mechanisms of adaptation, mechanisms that, through abuse, have become dependent on the chemicals in cigarette smoke to help them perform normally. That readjustment, which the body experiences as withdrawal symptoms, is an essential step in restoring the body's mechanisms for preserving its tendency to health. Indeed, it has been shown that heavy smokers who quit greatly reduce their health risks in the short term and, in time, can completely eliminate the risks.

So, as in all the other lifestyle factors considered so far, smoking is one of those easy choices associated with degeneration of the body's ability to stay healthy. The hard choice is to quit. Later, when we turn to the spiritual perspectives of health management, we will develop some strategies for making such hard choices and sticking to them.

Caffeine

Caffeine is the most commonly used of a group of substances I call the "stress drugs." Included in this group of drugs are chemicals related to amphetamine, such as amphetamine itself and some popular over-the-counter decongestant and diet drugs (phenylpropanolamine; pseudoephedrine). Also included among the stress drugs are the methylated xanthines, of which caffeine is a representative. These are all stimulant drugs with substantial power to alter metabolic control.

The responses such drugs provoke in the body are physiologically equivalent to reactions identified with the experience of stress.[7] I will say more about stress in a later chapter; here I would simply like to introduce the effects caused by the stress drugs, specifically caffeine.

The stress response is the body's prime mechanism for adapting to a need for physical reaction. It prepares the body to respond physically by increasing such functions as heart rate, blood pressure and muscle reactivity. Often called the fight-or-flight response, this series of reactions is a component of the body's normal mechanism of survival adaptation. Of course, a little stress response is always necessary because the body is always engaged in some amount of basal activity. But drugs are never required to stimulate the mechanism to function. In fact, to use drugs to provoke the mechanism when the body has no need for physical reaction is to abuse the system. Unnecessary drug-induced physical response is expressed in the body as one or more of a whole series of unpleasant reactions: nervousness, tension, gastrointestinal disturbance, headache and so on.

The stress drugs thus abuse the body's mechanisms of adaptation by provoking them into activity when no activity is required. When such drugs are consumed in substantial amounts on a regular basis, two stages of potentially harmful effects can occur. In the initial stage, the individual experiences regular occurrence of the symptoms of an unwanted stress response. Then, if abuse is continued, the body's adaptation mechanisms become altered so that the presence of the drug becomes absolutely essential for proper functioning of the system. Intake of the drug is then required just to get the stress response up to what is needed for maintaining the body's normal functions. At this stage, for example, an individual may say, "I can't get going in the morning until I've had at least two cups of coffee." It's a form of dependence, the substitution of a drug for a normal physiological function.

Although other stress drugs are commonly available, primarily in over-the-counter diet preparations and as decongestants in cold formulas, caffeine is by far the most abused of the drugs that promote unwanted stress response. Americans consume one-third of a pound of caffeine per year for every man, woman and child in the population. Most of this is consumed in coffee, tea and cola drinks, although caffeine is also used widely in pain formulas, diet drugs and the so-called stay-alert tablets. In addition, cocoa contains a closely related compound, called theobromine, which can provoke a similar stimulant effect in the body.

Regrettably, many people have the idea that because these drugs are consumed in natural products (such as coffee or chocolate), their use somehow becomes more acceptable. I have asked many people who are regular coffee drinkers if they had ever taken, or would consider taking, one of the stay-alert drugs. The answer is almost always an indignant and emphatic no. Yet the most popular stay-alert preparation contains just 100 milligrams of caffeine, *less* than the amount in one cup of coffee. It's amazing how many people will criticize someone who takes a couple of stay-alert pills to keep from falling asleep at the wheel, yet who think nothing of downing several cups of coffee themselves before they start for work in the morning!

An average cup of regular coffee provides about 110 milligrams of caffeine. If you drink three cups of coffee, the amount of caffeine consumed from them would make a tablet the size of a regular aspirin. To compare the other common sources of the drug, an average cup of tea contains about 90 milligrams of caffeine per cup. Cola drinks range from 20 to 55 milligrams per 12-ounce serving. Hot chocolate averages about 120 milligrams of theobromine per cup.[8]

At the levels provided by one serving of most of these products, caffeine is a very active stimulant. As the intake increases, noticeable symptoms become common: nausea, nervousness, insomnia and diuresis (increased urine flow). At higher average intakes (say, above 500 milligrams per day), the risk of developing cardiac arhythmias (irregular heartbeat) is very high.

Caffeine is a powerful, stress-inducing drug, particularly at the intake levels that have become common in our society. By itself it can provide a significant stress burden to one's life. When that burden is added to other origins of stress that people commonly experience, it can become the last straw in a person's total accumulation of unwanted stress. Caffeine intakes that lead to such stress burdens are the consequence of a lifestyle choice. If we want to eliminate that unwanted stress from our lives, we have to choose to alter our lifestyles either to avoid intake of the drug altogether, or to moderate our intake to more tolerable levels.

7 Physical Inactivity

*T*HE HUMAN BODY WAS NOT BUILT FOR LEISURE. IT WAS BUILT FOR physical labor. When we were invested by God at birth with a tendency toward good health, an implicit requirement for the preservation of that tendency was that our bodies be put to work. The only way health can be maintained at its birth potential is for the body to be challenged continually with regular physical activity.

Until the twentieth century, such physical activity was not necessarily a matter of choice; it was a matter of survival. For all but a small fraction of the population, survival was achieved by the sweat of one's brow. Now leisure is regarded as a way of life, and physical activity as something to be disdained. We don't walk anywhere if we can possibly avoid it. We wouldn't think of taking the stairs in a public building (if we could find them). We spend much of our incomes for labor-saving devices to assure that our evasion of exercise will be as complete as possible. Many people spend more time per week watching television than their ancestors spent laboring for a week's pay. Progress has made leisure an essential part of the good life in modern society, and we have flocked in great numbers to that choice.

The health consequences of a mass embrace of sedentary life have been, and will continue to be, disastrous. People who remain physically inactive are at much greater risk for cardiovascular disease (CVD) than those who exercise regularly. Because physical inactivity helps promote overweight, it contributes to all of the health risks that overweight promotes. Because physical activity preserves fitness generally, failure to exercise can be a significant factor in degeneration of our bodies' resistance to other disease.

Sometimes one gets the impression that a major reawakening to the importance of exercise has occurred. There is little evidence, however, that any substantial change has taken place in the exercise practices of most North Americans. The small minority who have made exercise a regular part of their lifestyles have received a lot of public attention recently, but they remain a small minority. For most, exercise is looked on as inconvenient, time-consuming and physically unpleasant. They opt for the easy choice and relax. They may buy an exercise bicycle or enroll at a neighborhood health club—and they may even give exercise a try—but few participate to the extent that their bodies require for minimum preservation of their health potential. Some try to fool themselves into thinking that a regular round of golf can be called exercise, even though they cover most of the distance in a golf cart. No, we haven't experienced a change in attitudes toward exercise. Rather, we're seeing a growth of a very profitable industry that supports the "exercise facade" behind which we hide while clinging to our love of leisure.

Challenge the Heart

To understand the importance of exercise we need a brief intro-
duction to exercise physiology. Muscular action is at the heart of
all physiological function in the human body. Even our basal
activities (those that continue when the body is at complete rest)
depend on muscular function. For example, although the tissues
of the brain or the liver contain no muscles themselves, they
cannot function without the benefit of muscular activity. They
need to be supplied with a constant flow of food and oxygen, and
to have their metabolic waste products removed. These essential
tasks are primarily the function of the cardiovascular system.

The heart is a muscle, a remarkable one. In an average person,
even at rest, the heart beats over 100 thousand times every day.
It moves a total volume of blood of almost 3,000 gallons daily.
Properly cared for, it can sustain that workload and much more,
without a rest, for seventy or eighty years or even longer. It was
not intended to be an organ of sloth. The minimal demands of
basal metabolism are not adequate to keep the heart in tune
physically. It needs heavier workloads on a regular basis to preserve its inborn potential. It will degenerate in functional ability
if it is not regularly challenged to operate up to its capabilities.
The way to create such a challenge is through physical activity.

We cannot consider exercise of the heart without considering
at the same time the exercise of other substantial muscle masses
in the body, those of the skeletal muscle system. We challenge
the heart by exercising the muscles we use to run, swim, dig,
cycle, lift or whatever other activity we engage in. In addition,
exercise has a general positive influence on body chemistry and
on the ability of the body to perform its other physiological
functions. A simple example is the improvement in serum cholesterol levels in people who exercise regularly.

For some people, notably the so-called body builders, challenging the skeletal muscles through exercise is an end in itself.

However, because our goal is not to build big muscles but to avoid the primary causes of degenerative disease, we have to look at muscular activity more as a means than an end. When we develop strategies for implementing a personal exercise program, we have to keep our priorities in mind. Our exercise activities must contribute ultimately and significantly to strengthening the cardiovascular system.

Let's assume that you are a sedentary but otherwise healthy adult, possibly a bit overweight, and interested in improving your chances for a long and healthy life. To accomplish that goal, you need to undertake a *regular* program of physical exercise—but *without killing yourself in the process*. The requirement that you survive the process adds another dimension, one of caution. If you are not *absolutely* certain of your present ability to increase your physical activity without endangering your health, two precautionary actions are highly recommended. They are advisable, in fact, even if you do feel capable.

First, submit yourself to examination by a physician, who will be able to test your present physical condition and assess your ability to withstand an increase in activity. Second, do your exercise, at least initially, under the supervision of a qualified professional. Your local YMCA, YWCA or health club offers exercise programs for virtually every level of ability and achievement, with professional supervision.

Aerobic Capacity
The first thing a sedentary person detects when exercise is attempted is a decided lack of endurance. Even a low level of exercise leads quickly to exhaustion. We quickly learn the meaning of "out of shape." The primary factor in our lack of endurance is something called *aerobic capacity*. The term *aerobic* has become a buzz word among fitness cultists but few people understand what it means. Even fewer understand what to do with it. The

term *aerobic* means *oxygen dependent*. To appreciate that definition, we need to know a little more about how the human body generates energy.

As in mechanical systems like an automobile, the body generates energy by "burning" fuel. The energy produced in that process permits the muscles to do work. Unlike an automobile engine, however, which can function only if it is provided with a constant flow of air (oxygen), the body has the capability of generating energy either in the presence or absence of oxygen. When energy is produced in the body with oxygen present, the process is called *aerobic* metabolism. When oxygen is absent, the energy metabolism is called *anaerobic* (oxygen independent).

Each of those processes offers certain advantages since the body is called on to do work under various conditions. Aerobic metabolism is highly fuel-efficient and can use both fat and carbohydrate as fuel. Anaerobic metabolism can use only carbohydrate as fuel, and it uses that fuel *twenty times less efficiently* than when oxygen is present. In anaerobic metabolism, lactic acid accumulates in the muscles, a primary cause of the muscle soreness experienced by people who try to do more physically than their bodies are prepared to sustain. You may ask why anaerobic metabolism is ever used, if it is so inefficient and produces such unpleasant side effects. The answer is that, in certain muscles under certain circumstances, oxygen is simply not available. That's what happens when we are out of breath. Literally, there is not enough oxygen to meet all our needs. But we don't die. Instead we keep going. That is because anaerobic metabolism allows for energy production that would otherwise be impossible. A prime goal in physical conditioning is to reduce the proportion of energy produced by anaerobic oxidation during exercise. That reduction is accomplished by developing what I called *aerobic capacity*.

Aerobic capacity is a measure of the body's ability to deliver oxygen to working muscles. That capacity is mainly a function of two systems: the respiratory system, which takes oxygen from the air and assimilates it into the blood, and the cardiovascular system, which delivers the oxygen to the tissues. If those systems function at very low efficiency because a sedentary lifestyle has allowed their capabilities to degenerate, your aerobic capacity will be very low. Under those conditions, even a little physical activity will overload the systems; your body will have to resort to anaerobic metabolism to support the activity, leading very quickly to exhaustion.

To increase aerobic capacity, the systems that contribute to it have to be challenged. The systematic process through which such challenges are implemented is called *conditioning.* However, not all exercise strategies necessarily provide significant challenges to the oxygen-delivery system. As a result, many efforts to achieve meaningful conditioning are really "exercises in futility."

Any amount of exercise is, of course, better than none. But unless the heart rate can be increased to a challenging level at regular intervals for reasonable periods of time, the exercise will do little toward cardiovascular conditioning. Some general standards are available for what constitutes a challenging heart rate and a reasonable exercise period, although you may want to seek professional advice before making that determination for yourself. Most authorities concur that we must exercise at least three times per week if it is to have any real value. As a rule of thumb, we can assume that a heart rate of 80 per cent of maximum, sustained for fifteen minutes, will constitute a reasonable challenge to the cardiovascular system. (To estimate your maximum heart rate, subtract your age from 220.)

Developing a Personal Program
The amount of workout time necessary for effective conditioning

depends to a great extent on your current physical condition. If you have been sedentary for a long while, you will certainly find that even a short exercise period (perhaps five minutes) is a significant challenge for you. Repeating your minimum workout at regular intervals (three to four times per week), will give you some improvement in your physical condition. Although that improvement may seem significant when measured against your poor starting condition, it will be relatively small when measured against what your condition should be to insure maximum health and longevity.

So, as your physical condition improves, it will be necessary to increase your total exercise challenge to assure progressive improvement in cardiovascular capacity. That increase can be effected by increasing exercise intensity or by increasing your workout time or both. Within the limits of individual capability, I tend to favor establishing a constant maximum challenge to heart rate (exercise intensity) as early in the program as possible and then increasing workout time as improved physical condition permits.

The type of exercise chosen is a matter of personal preference and personal physical limitations. Not everyone has to be a jogger to develop good cardiovascular conditioning. Swimming and cycling, for example, are also excellent ways to challenge the major muscle masses. Walking can be a good way to introduce yourself to conditioning and to establish an exercise discipline, but few people can or want to walk vigorously enough to produce an effective cardiovascular challenge. Calisthenics are somewhat better, but people seldom want to spend the time necessary to make that kind of exercise useful in conditioning. Recreational sports such as racquetball and tennis can be useful in cardiovascular conditioning, if played *regularly* and at a reasonable intensity.

I abandoned my own sedentary life when I learned that a high-school classmate had suffered a heart attack. I started by skipping rope. Within a few months, though, I found I could not maintain a sufficient cardiovascular challenge without becoming bored silly. I took up running, starting with about eight-minute workouts four times per week. Now I run three miles every day at a fairly challenging pace to maintain the conditioning I have developed.

One important thing to recognize as you undertake a conditioning program is that it is not necessary to sustain the exercise in order to sustain an elevated heart rate. In fact, even for athletes in training, exercise carried out in "intervals" is much more effective for aerobic conditioning than is sustained exercise. The logic behind that fact is simple. The kind of exercise that can build a heart rate to challenging levels requires, because of its high intensity, a significant amount of anaerobic metabolism, particularly for people in poor physical condition. After even a few minutes of such exercise, the average out-of-shape individual will be exhausted, discouraged and sore—a prime candidate for dropping out. But such consequences are completely unnecessary. It's possible to implement effective aerobic conditioning without having to suffer exhaustion, and without *ever* experiencing sore muscles. All it takes is a little common sense.

Let's say that, for you, an 80 per cent maximum heart rate is 140 beats per minute. If you exercise for a short interval (twenty to thirty seconds) at a level that will take the heart rate to 145, and then rest until it decreases to 135, repeating this exercise/ rest pattern as your heart rate dictates, some interesting advantages will accrue. First, you will maintain the target average heart rate of 140 for the desired workout period. Second, the rest intervals will allow recovery to occur, decreasing the total production of lactic acid and accelerating its removal from the muscles. Exercise conducted in this way can give a high level of cardiovascular conditioning without the unpleasant effects that cause so many beginners to quit.

Because of frequent confusion, I would like to clarify the difference between "aerobic exercise" and "aerobic conditioning." Exercise is considered to be aerobic when it can be completely supported by the present ability of the body to deliver oxygen. Obviously then, for most people, this kind of exercise has to be of *very low intensity*. Thus aerobic exercise is of little value for aerobic conditioning. It can be useful for maintaining an already developed aerobic capacity, once it has been achieved, but it has none of the right elements to promote conditioning in the first place. To be considered aerobic, the exercise cannot provoke a significant amount of anaerobic metabolism. Yet the kinds of workloads required to challenge the oxygen-delivery system have to be significantly anaerobic, or they won't do the job.

How can you tell whether exercise is aerobic or anaerobic? That's easy. If you end up huffing and puffing, the exercise has been significantly anaerobic, because the panting is necessary to pay back the oxygen debt that the muscles built up when they didn't get enough oxygen to do their work. Aerobic exercise can be sustained without such extreme demands on respiration. You don't need to be an expert to know when your exercise is aerobic and when it is not. You may have signed up for a class called "aerobic dance" but, if you end up huffing and puffing, it's not really aerobic. Don't forget, though, that if you don't do some huffing and puffing, you're not going to gain much in the way of preventive conditioning.

One other perspective on exercise may be useful to you, particularly if you are concerned about the role of exercise in weight loss. First of all, it should be evident that the kind of exercise that is best for conditioning the cardiovascular system is of limited value for weight loss. Why? Because that kind of exercise is significantly anaerobic, and anaerobic metabolism *uses only carbohydrate fuel*. Successful weight loss uses up fat and, if you want to burn body fat, *the exercise has to be aerobic.* But aerobic exercise is fundamentally of low intensity, so it burns fuel slowly. It is also very fuel-efficient, so it takes a lot of exercise to burn up a few calories of body fat.

For example, I have heard people justify a big, rich dessert at dinner by declaring "Tomorrow I'm going to get more exercise." They probably have no idea how *much* exercise is required to burn up the calories in that dessert. A generous serving of apple pie ala mode contains about 550 calories. To burn off that many calories means walking six miles or doing calisthenics for several hours. Few people are willing to undertake that kind of exercise obligation just to work off the calories from one dessert. For most people the best exercise for losing weight is simply pushing away from the table. They still should be exercising regularly, however, for preventive conditioning.

Implementation of an effective physical conditioning program requires commitment. Conditioning exercise has to be regular; it has to become a permanent part of our lifestyles. That means a significant investment in time and energy. Yet, if we use common sense and do it right, we may be surprised to find how easy it is.

8 Stress

*I*N TRYING TO UNDERSTAND STRESS, WE ARE DEALING ALMOST TO-tally with opinion rather than with experimentally verified facts. We know what stress is, but we have no research data on what causes its unwanted occurrence in people's lives. Yet we need to understand its origins if we hope to eliminate it. So we speculate on what causes stress and base our strategies for control on those speculations. Of course, if our speculations are wrong, the strategies for control will be inadequate.

Since stress education in our culture is failing to stem a rising tide of stress-related problems, it would be pretty safe to say that most current speculations on the causes of unwanted stress are wrong. That is because those speculations have not been firmly founded on common sense. Someone once asked me how I had arrived at the details of my philosophy on prevention of un-wanted stress. I replied that I started with the definition of stress (found in any physiology textbook), insisted that my conclusions obey the laws of common sense and then just followed my nose. Over the years a lot of people have benefited from a willingness to follow common sense in preventing their unwanted stress. In the following pages I have tried to summarize that common sense.

My work in stress education has led me to two fundamental conclusions about responsible health management. First, stress is probably the influence at work in modern society that is most damaging to health. Second, that influence is *totally preventable.* In all my work in health education, I find no aspect more important than helping people learn how to prevent unwanted stress.

Stress is a common denominator in virtually all health-threatening lifestyles. It is frequently a major contributing factor to dietary practices promoting degenerative disease. It is often the major contributor to substance abuse. By itself it can cause such common disorders as ulcers and irritable bowel syndrome. It may be the single most significant risk factor in cardiovascular disease (CVD). Many authorities believe that its degenerative influence on body resistance contributes materially to susceptibility to other diseases—from the common cold to cancer.

Why is stress so much greater a problem today than it was at the turn of the century? The consensus would be that life today in the Western world is much more complex and that coping with the pressures of life in modern society requires more stress. That consensus, though, is *completely wrong.* Yet it identifies the problem: we do not understand what stress is; we do not understand who or what is responsible for its existence; and thus we have absolutely no idea how to go about eliminating its unwanted presence.

That lack of awareness is all the more regrettable because it is being actively fed from misconceptions promoted by those who claim to provide a solution. Those misconceptions, which I term "the stress myth," actually do more to perpetuate unwanted stress in our culture than any other single factor. To deal with stress, we must first deal with "the stress myth."

Stress and Excess Stress

Stress is *not* something that our environment imposes on us. It is our personal reaction to that environment. Stress is a human survival mechanism, a *physical* response, intended solely to prepare the body *physically* to deal with its circumstances.[1] The progress and extent of those preparations can be measured specifically by certain physical changes that occur during the stress response: an increase in heart rate and blood pressure, changes in blood flow (to favor the muscles and brain), increases in muscle tone and nerve excitability, and increases in the availability of fuel for the brain, to name just a few. It should be evident that all of these physiological reactions serve one common purpose: to equip the body for *decisive physical reaction.* The fundamental purpose of the response is to insure survival by preparing the body to take appropriate action.

Everyone puts the stress response to use for that purpose every day. Stress insures your survival by promoting quick reactions whenever the unexpected happens. But not all such physical preparations necessarily have specific survival value. Any increase in physical activity requires a stress response to facilitate the body's preparations for the activity. Thus, exercise necessarily causes stress. Athletes and people whose employment requires intensive physical labor spend a lot of time under high levels of stress. From this perspective it takes much more stress to be a ditch digger than to run General Motors.

The fundamental problem with stress in modern society is not that stress exists. It should be clear by now that it *has* to exist if the human race is to survive. Problems occur only when stress exists at the wrong times and in the wrong amounts. What is an appropriate time? Any time that the body has an *actual need* for *immediate physical reaction*. What is an appropriate amount of stress? The amount necessary to prepare the body to deal adequately with the circumstances with which it is confronted— *and no more than that*. The stress response is excessive when it goes beyond the actual physical need. That unnecessary stress, which I call excess stress, is what people typically identify as the unpleasant consequences of what they usually call stress.

So the first thing to do in coming to grips with unwanted stress in life is to learn to distinguish between necessary or appropriate stress and excess stress. Most of us are unaware of any appropriate stress, at least until after our body's requirement for it has passed. Athletes, for example, normally don't sense the existence of stress even when its levels are very high. They suffer no ill effects from its presence. They just do their work, content in the consequences of their stress—that is, in the ability of their bodies to meet the physical demands of competition. With no excess stress at those times, they experience no unpleasant consequences.

Here is the key: there is never any unpleasantness associated with necessary stress. Unpleasant sensations are due solely to excess stress. In fact, we can define excess stress in those specific terms: if the stress experienced is unpleasant, then the response is excessive to the body's physical needs at the time.

To illustrate the difference between appropriate stress and excess stress, let's look at the reactions of two different people required to deal with identical situations. Mr. Adams and Mr. Baker are both design engineers for a manufacturing company. A problem has come up in the design of a critical project. Two components have to be re-engineered. The requirements of the two tasks are equivalent. The two engineers are each given one of the components and told by their supervisors that the new designs must be finished in four hours.

How much stress is needed to prepare the body adequately to deal with the physical and physiological demands of these projects? A little. But not very much. As he sits down at his desk to confront the problem before him, Mr. Adams produces just enough stress to allow him to deal with its demands, but no more than that. Mr. Baker, on the other hand, has a massive stress response as he contemplates the time and performance pressures placed on him. He, like Mr. Adams, needs only a little stress to do the job before him. But he produces a very large amount, much more than he needs. Mr. Adams has no excess stress. Mr. Baker has almost nothing but excess stress.

Who is likely to do the better job, and why? Not Mr. Baker. That excess stress is not only going to be useless to him, it could be disastrous to his performance. Stress is a very powerful regulator in the human body. Most of us have heard stories of people who in times of crisis have shown superhuman strength in dealing with a situation. That's what stress is capable of doing in the interest of survival.

But suppose our circumstances don't call for any significant physical reaction. If enough stress is still produced to prompt superhuman effort, that excess stress can be just as powerful in causing damage. The fact that it is so universally regarded as unpleasant, and that people so often resort to extreme behaviors to avoid it, gives testimony to its power. Further, it may be the direct cause of many of the fatal heart attacks that occur in this country.[2] It can also prompt people to worry holes in their own stomachs (ulcers). You can imagine, then, that with such destructive power at work in him, Mr. Baker is not going to be well equipped to complete the job before him. The right amount of stress is good. More is never better.

Mr. Adams had an appropriate stress response. Mr. Baker had a response dominated by excess stress. Yet they had equivalent tasks, they were equally competent and they had the same deadline. What was the difference? The difference was in how each chose to deal with the circumstances before him.

Thus we return to that all-important element of personal choice. It is at this point that we come directly into conflict with the stress myth. The myth would have us believe that unwanted stress is not a matter of choice but of circumstances. The myth tells us that stress is the result of things that happen in the world and that we are the victims of those happenings. According to the myth, we have no choice in our experience of stress. Such a point of view can be comforting for those who wish to avoid taking responsibility for their stress, but it is completely contrary to what we know about stress and how it occurs.

One of the tools used to perpetuate the stress myth is a document called "The Social Readjustment Rating Scale."[3] It is a list of life events to which values have been assigned, indicating the supposed tendency of each event to provoke stress. You have probably seen that scale, or variations of it, printed in books or magazine articles on stress, or perhaps used as a party game. Stress-myth practitioners try to use it to estimate the total amount of stress people have. Thus, if a person has experienced several of the high-scoring events on the list (death in the family, divorce, unemployment), he or she is supposedly fated to a life of unwanted stress, and nothing can be done about it. Some even suggest that a person's chance of maintaining health will depend on one's score. According to them, a high score means that we are inevitably destined to get physically sick. What colossal nonsense.

I call that insidious document the permission slip because the only thing it does is give us permission to avoid responsibility for our own stress. In the process, of course, it takes away any possibility of personal control over the stress we would like to prevent. No matter what the myth tells us, and whether or not we choose to believe it, the occurrence of unwanted stress is *always* our own personal responsibility. Let me be clear. We do not always choose what events will happen to us. But we do choose how we will respond to those events. And it is the response that can cause excess stress, not the events. Thus, unwanted stress will be prevented only when we choose for it not to occur. No matter how much we may be inclined to reject the truth of it, we are 100 per cent in charge of our own reactions to the world in which we live.

The Stressor Within

This is a difficult fact for most people to accept. Conditioned by the stress myth, we have come to believe that the events of life are responsible for our stress. People who have jobs that place them under pressure blame the jobs. Those who have conflict in their family lives blame the relationship or other family members. If life has been particularly difficult and I react with stress, it's easy to convince myself that the circumstances are responsible for my stress.

Many use the term *stressor* to describe those outside influences to which people assign responsibility for their unwanted stress. Thus, from the stress myth we get a picture of a world full of stressors just waiting to provoke stress in the people they encounter. That view promotes the idea that the only way to get rid of the stress is to get rid of the stressor. So people spend a tremendous amount of time and effort trying to do just that: eliminate the stressor.

The problem is that there is no such thing as a stressor out there in the world; we generate them from our reactions to the world. All of that time and effort is being spent trying to eliminate something that *doesn't even exist*. It's no wonder, then, that we are having a difficult time dealing with our stress.

To put the true origins of stress into a manageable perspective, let's apply some common sense to what we already know about stress—what it is and how it occurs—and about the world in which we live. What can we say, with objectivity and some amount of certainty, about the world around us?

What we know for sure is that the world is a vast source of information. That information does not come to us with ready-made interpretations. It is strictly neutral. For example, if you were to turn a mouse loose in a room full of people, from the purely objective standpoint the mouse exists only as an item of information. The information relates to size, shape, color, movement characteristics and so on. Those same items of information are transmitted, without deviation, to every person in the room. The information constitutes the *reality* of the situation.

But not everyone in the room deals with that reality in the same way. One person shrieks and leaps onto the nearest chair. Another person's only reaction is a slight chuckle, contemplating the prospect of someone being "treed" by a harmless creature of such minute proportions. The reality of the situation was no different for either of them. The difference was in how they personally interpreted that reality. The first person reacted with stress. The second did not, so clearly the mouse was not a stressor for that person. But was it a stressor for the first one? Of course not. It remained nothing but a source of information for both of them. The stressor was the first person's interpretation of that information.

So, stressors do not exist out in the world. They exist, when they do exist, solely as a result of a person's interpretation of the realities of that world. They are matters of choice, not matters of fact. Does this mean, then, that one individual's stress in reaction to a mouse is inappropriate, simply because that person misinterprets the reality of the circumstances? Not at all. When people think they are facing a threat, they react every bit the same as if the threat were real. They aren't in physical danger, but they think they are—and that is what's important. But, whether the stress is appropriate or not, it is essential to understand that it *always* occurs by choice—it is an *elective reaction* to whatever one's reality is interpreted to be.

Consider another situation. Mr. Carson has been working hard to make a major sale, one that would mean a substantial commission and the possibility of promotion. But he has just been informed that his hoped-for sale went to someone else. Now he sits alone at his desk. He is hurt and angry. His heart rate and blood pressure are elevated. He is tense and on edge. He has a headache and his stomach is upset. He is having a stress response, a substantial one.

But what is his actual need for physical response in the present circumstances? Virtually none. How much of his stress is excess stress? Almost all of it. Remember, stress has one and only one purpose: to prepare the body *physically* to deal with some threat to its stability. If no physical threat exists (real or imagined), then the stress is always inappropriate. It will be excess stress and it will provoke the destructive consequences which invariably result from the misdirection of this powerful influence.

Why did Mr. Carson choose to have a stress response when it was so inappropriate to his circumstances? The answer to that question, of course, is the key to the prevention of unwanted stress. He had an inappropriate stress response because he made an erroneous interpretation. He perceived incorrectly the reality of his circumstances. He interpreted that reality as a threat. Did he consider it a physical threat? No. He didn't view it as an assault on his physical stability. Rather, he saw it as a threat to his *emotional* stability. Yet the body has only one mechanism for dealing with threats to its stability, and that mechanism is physical. Excess stress typically occurs when an event is interpreted as a threat to emotional stability (a stressor, if you will), and the body reacts to that stressor in the only way it knows how—with stress. However, because emotional threats require no physical response, the stress that results from them is *always inappropriate.* Clearly, then, if we want to prevent the occurrence of excess stress, we need to know something about how threats to emotional stability can happen and what can be done to prevent them.

To describe our emotional nature, I use a model called the stability structure. I define it as the total of all the principles, ideals, standards and values by which each of us establishes his or her own self-image and through which each person determines how that self-concept is affected by reality. I call it the stability structure because its purpose is to preserve emotional stability whenever we are confronted with potentially unstabilizing life events. It is basically an interpreter. It takes information from the world and interprets its influence on our concepts of personal identity. If the interpretation confirms or enhances self-image, stability is maintained. If the interpretation diminishes that image, emotional instability occurs and the body reacts with stress. Inappropriate, excess stress.

In simple terms, then, unnecessary and unwanted stress occurs because we interpret life events in ways that adversely affect self-image. Such interpretations are strictly a matter of *personal choice,* because both the self-image and the interpretations based on that image are strictly products of personal choice. A self-image is exactly what the name suggests—a personal opinion. It is not a matter of fact. It is a matter of belief. With that fundamental truth, we come to the core of the problem with unwanted stress. Excess stress occurs not because life is full of threatening events but because flaws exist in our *belief systems,* flaws that allow such events to diminish our concepts of self.

Unwanted stress is not eliminated by attempts to change reality. Reality is what it is; perception is what has to change. Unnecessary stress has its origin in flawed perception and will be prevented only when the flaw is corrected. This puts a new and different perspective on the business of personal stress management. All these years we've been attempting to get rid of our unwanted stress by fighting reality, avoiding reality or trying to live with our unhealthy reactions to reality. Now, we find that all we have to do to prevent the stress is to amend the flaws in our self-images that led to faulty perceptions of that reality.

But is it never appropriate to attempt to alter our situations? If I am unemployed, shouldn't I try to find another job? If I'm getting bad grades, shouldn't I try to put more study time in my schedule? If I am overweight, shouldn't I try to eat better? Obviously, yes. But I am not concerned here with what decisions to make. I am concerned with stress—and how to prevent unwanted stress *while* I am trying to improve my situation. It may be very appropriate to change our circumstances, but not as a means of eliminating excess stress.

What Motivates Stress?

As in any kind of trouble-shooting, stress prevention requires that one first locate and identify the problem (here, the flaw in one's self-image), then do whatever is necessary to correct it. To help you do that, I would like to introduce a powerful trouble-shooting technique. I call the technique stress analysis. Its purpose is to help you understand the motives behind human behavior—your own behavior and that of other people. First let's see how it is used to assess someone else's behavior.

A problem that frequently comes up in groups I work with is what I've come to call "The Strange Case of the Manipulating Mother-in-Law." The behavior in this case takes various forms, but a typical scenario is a mother-in-law/daughter-in-law relationship in which the mother-in-law has to be in control of circumstances at all times. When the daughter-in-law is the visitor, she is not allowed to do anything. The mother-in-law has everything under tight personal control. Further, when the mother-in-law is the visitor, she still takes over. The daughter-in-law finds herself taking orders in her own home. Those things the mother-in-law can't control directly, she attempts to manipulate through an endless stream of advice and not-so-subtle hints.

Why does the mother-in-law behave this way? The daughter-in-law feels it's because her mother-in-law doesn't like her, considers her to be a moron who can't do anything on her own and believes the daughter-in-law is not good enough for her son. The younger woman has attributed ill will as the overriding motive behind the older woman's behavior, and has chosen her own reaction to the mother-in-law on the basis of that assessment. Is it an accurate assessment? Most often it is not.

The need to control is an expression of what could be called stress-motivated behavior. It is an effort on the part of an individual to avoid the unpleasantness of unwanted stress by trying to manipulate the events of life. The controller incorrectly views the world as the source of his or her stress, and desperately tries to manipulate the world to avoid the excess stress. Of course, such manipulations are always futile because the world is never responsible for the stress. The unpleasant stress is caused by a faulty personal perception of that world. In addition, stress-motivated behavior is virtually always destructive in outcome, not only because of its failure in purpose but also because it attempts to manipulate reality. When that reality affects the lives of other people, conflict usually results.

The purpose of stress analysis is not to assess the *consequences* of stress-motivated behavior, however, but to establish its *motive*. What is the mother-in-law's motive in behaving the way she does? Survival. Emotional survival. She is trying, in the only way she knows how, to avoid the devastating effects that are inevitably caused by her own faulty perception of reality. Her perception is almost guaranteed to make a shambles of her self-image and provoke a substantial and decidedly unpleasant stress response. Because she is unaware of the true cause of that stress, her efforts to control the stress are directed toward what she *thinks* is its cause: the world in which she lives; the life events she is experiencing.

The motivating logic of a person who has a need to control is simple. It says, "If I can only get my world, and the people in it, to be the way I want them to be, then I won't have to perceive that world in ways that make me think less of myself." There we have the solution to "The Strange Case of the Manipulating Mother-in-Law." Like a drowning person struggling to stay afloat, she is just trying to survive to preserve stability.

The problem most of us have in dealing with such behavior is reflected in the daughter-in-law's reaction. Typically, people want to evaluate such behavior on the basis of its wisdom and its consequences rather than on its motive. Certainly, if survival is the mother-in-law's goal, her attempts at manipulation are not wise. The consequences of her actions are certainly anything but constructive. But neither of these facts is of any importance in stress analysis. The only important thing to understand is why she does it. In this situation, as in the vast majority of such cases, the motive behind the manipulation is a desire to avoid the unpleasant experience of unwanted stress.

Stress analysis enables us to attribute a nonthreatening motive to behavior. It does not in any way require that we approve the behavior. It merely gives us the opportunity to understand what's behind it. In our dealings with other people, stress analysis allows us to avoid reacting to their actions and helps us learn to respond to the fears and uncertainties that motivate their actions.

For example, the daughter-in-law can learn to appreciate that the mother-in-law actually feels threatened by her son's wife. Then the younger woman, instead of reacting with hurt feelings and anger, can respond in ways that will diminish the uncertainty that the mother-in-law feels. The alternative, of course, is for the young wife herself to feel threatened by her mother-in-law's manipulations and respond with her *own* manipulations, intended to change her concept of reality so that *she* doesn't have to feel stressed. Such defensive interaction is typical of interpersonal conflict, reflecting a joint inability or unwillingness to acknowledge what really motivates people to behave the way they do.

Conditional Self-Image

The process of stress analysis is essentially no different when used to help us understand our own actions. Of course, it is more difficult because we have become skilled over the years in overlooking or misinterpreting our own motives. But if we're serious about preventing our own experience of unwanted stress, we're going to have to learn how to do it. We need to find the flaws in our own personalities which provoke us to stress when no stress is necessary.

The key is to find the best time to look for flaws. Obviously, this is usually when our flaws are expressing themselves, when we experience unwanted stress. It is at those times that we need to stop and ask why. Why do I react to this particular situation with stress when none is needed? What is there about the circumstances with which I am confronted that compels me to respond by diminishing my concept of self? Where is the flaw in my identity structure that permits a neutral life event to be interpreted as a stressor?

For example, go back to Mr. Carson who had excess stress when he failed to make an important sale. If at the time he was feeling stress he had stopped to analyze his response, he would have discovered something in his stability structure that declared, "I have value as a person only when I succeed in my work." A corollary principle declares, "If I don't succeed, I'm nothing."

Mr. Baker, the uptight engineer, operated on a similar principle. Only he didn't even wait to fail to put it to work. He had an unnecessary stress response just contemplating failure.

What about the mother-in-law? Her stability structure contains a slightly different "conditional." It says, "I can consider myself to be of value as a person only when things are the way I want them to be." Every time you have an unnecessary and unwanted stress response, it will be the result of a similar conditional in your identity structure, imposing restrictions on your ability to accept your own value as a human being.

All of these conditionals represent flaws. Why? Because your self-image should not be subject to influence by the events you experience in life. When you say, "I am less valuable as a person if . . ." or "I am less valuable as a person when . . . ," you are allowing your circumstances to dictate your identity. But it's *your* identity. You can make it absolutely anything you want. *The flaw is in granting to circumstances the prerogative to make your identity something other than what you want.*

How do you eliminate the flaw? By changing the way you establish your identity. How do you establish *your* identity? What do you use as the basis for your self-image? Can you create an image that has no flaws? As you ponder these questions, let me remind you of several essential facts. Your self-image is *yours* and *yours alone.* No matter what basis you may use for that image, no matter what outside information you may accept in establishing it, it is still totally yours and totally under your control. It is not permanent because you can change it any time you want. You are the only one in charge of its existence and of its characteristics. There should be no reason, then, why that image could not be perfect—no reason, that is, except one: a tendency to believe that you can be a better image-maker than God.

When God created you in his image, he placed his stamp of approval on you. As he did when he created Adam and Eve in that same image, he stood back and said, "It is very good." He declared unequivocally that you are special. Quite apart from your physical appearance, intellectual ability, family heritage or current circumstances, you are *somebody*. And what do you do with that amazing gift? You cast it aside, saying, "No, that's not completely true. I'm only somebody if . . . I'm only somebody when . . . Otherwise I'm nobody."

If you put yourself into the image-making business, you will experience a lot of unwanted stress when the ifs and whens and otherwises raise havoc with that image. To eliminate *all* of that unwanted stress, you only have to do one simple thing. Get out of the image-making business.

If you will accept God's image, without question and without reservation, the basis for all of your undesirable stress will be eliminated. The image of God is completely unassailable. It cannot be diminished by "powers and principalities"; it cannot be devalued by "things seen or unseen." It makes you into *somebody special*—no ifs, whens or buts.

Accepting God's image is a choice. It should be an easy choice —but obviously it isn't because so few people seem willing to make it their choice. The world is populated with people who, whatever their spiritual confessions, enthusiastically substitute their own conditional images for the true image of God. Then they strive to endure the unnecessary stress that inevitably goes with such substitution.

So we must look at the choice of image in the same way we have approached other lifestyle choices. The hard choice is to go with God. The other choice is to go one's own way, suffering the physical, emotional and spiritual consequences of misguided self-sufficiency.

9 Spiritual Perspectives on Staying Well

WHAT DOES SCRIPTURE TEACH ABOUT COMMITMENT *IN* Christian living? How do these teachings apply to the management of personal health? My answer to these questions is divided into four parts, each looking at the subject from a different perspective. The first section relates to *temptation,* the second to *promises,* the third to *dedication* and the fourth to *faith.* Overall, I have a whole-person perspective which views human health as multidimensional. That is, I view our physical identity to always be in dynamic interaction with an emotional identity and a spiritual identity.

The whole-person approach to understanding human health is by no means new. But a variety of definitions are developing as it once again becomes popular. Secular thinkers, of course, want to define it in such a way that *spiritual* does not have to be interpreted as requiring belief in God. Some eliminate the spiritual identity altogether when they describe the whole person. Even among Christians, there is not a consensus about the interrelationships of the physical, emotional and spiritual. Much of the popular Christian understanding of whole-person health relates to what one might call spiritual intervention, the healing of disease as a direct result of concerted acts of faith.

Without hesitation, I will assert my conviction that such healings do occur, and my belief that faith is a key factor in their occurrence. Our discussion here, however, is not about healing but about prevention. When we apply the whole-person concept to the prevention of disease, a somewhat different picture emerges.

Commitment and Compromise

As we have seen, disease prevention is basically a two-step process: (1) identify the cause; (2) eliminate it. One point of view among Christians is that human disease is caused by a direct act of Satan. They note that when Jesus healed a woman of a crippling infirmity, he said she was "bound by Satan" for eighteen years (Lk 13:16). Or they use Paul's description of his own "thorn in the flesh" as "a messenger of Satan" (2 Cor 12:7).

Yet the suggestion that Satan plays a universal role in the cause of human infirmity seems impossible to reconcile with another healing by Jesus. When Jesus was asked by his disciples what caused the condition of a man born blind, he said it was "that the works of God might be made manifest in him" (Jn 9:3).

Clearly, Jesus didn't always consider Satan to be directly responsible for disease. And, frankly, I don't believe we can justifiably hold Satan responsible as the direct cause of the degenerative diseases we have been considering. That is not to say that he has no part in the occurrence of those diseases. I am merely contending that he does not intervene directly in the body's normal tendency toward good health. Rather, I see his role as that of tempter, enticing individuals to make lifestyle choices that lead to degeneration. Perhaps you are familiar with the classic satire on Satan by C. S. Lewis, *The Screwtape Letters*. Lewis perceptively described the work of Satan in letters of instruction from a senior-grade devil, Screwtape, to his nephew Wormwood, a junior tempter with direct responsibility for the corruption of one human. In the following excerpt, Screwtape gives advice specifically on how lifestyle choices relate to physical well-being —and to further temptation:

> Keep your man in a condition of false spirituality. Never let him notice the medical aspect. Keep him wondering what pride or lack of faith has delivered him into your hands when a simple enquiry into what he has been eating or drinking for the last twenty-four hours would show him whence your ammunition comes and thus enable him by a very little abstinence to imperil your lines of communication.[1]

As a culture we have progressed from few lifestyle options, most of which promoted man's inborn tendency to health, to a multitude of options, many promoting degeneration of that tendency. Today's lifestyle choices can be either good or bad. How do we select among them? Often we select in ignorance. But is ignorance an acceptable excuse? For some people, such as the still primitive cultures of the world, it has to be. But, then, they have almost no incidence of the degenerative diseases that plague "civilized" peoples.

For Christians, that fact may trigger a long train of thought leading back to the Garden of Eden. Could it be true that when societies were more directly dependent on God and his creation for their sustenance, their lifestyle choices were much more consistent with preserving a tendency toward health? Did God in his wisdom give them almost no other alternatives? Obviously, primitive people are susceptible to disease and are not exempt from being assaulted by wild animals or unfriendly humans. But they seem not to suffer the degenerative physical consequences of bad choices leading to cardiovascular disease, diabetes and the like.

Progress, of itself, has not been the cause of degeneration in that tendency. It's just that progress has substituted human self-sufficiency for the wisdom of God, and the exercise of that self-sufficiency has been found wanting. But progress doesn't keep us from following God's creation wisdom. Today the preservation of health is eminently possible. All it requires is a reidentification of human purpose with the wisdom of God—in other words, a responsible exercise of Christian decision making.

That responsibility, of course, is constantly subject to subversion by temptation. The dictionary defines the word *tempt* like this: "To entice to what is wrong by promise of pleasure or gain." Of course, we can mentally reduce Satan to a kind of mythical construct that makes entertaining fiction but nothing more. Or we can take the same position as C. S. Lewis, that the Evil One actually takes advantage of every opportunity to subvert God's purposes and lead us into life choices that promote personal destruction. The unpleasant but unavoidable conclusion I draw is that submission to temptation is the primary force behind the degenerative health effects observed in today's civilized cultures. Whether or not you believe that Satan had a hand in prompting that submission, you can see that he will hug himself with joy over its ultimate consequences.

What constitutes temptation? If we are tempted when we are enticed "to what is wrong," how do we determine what is wrong? How can we put "pleasure or gain" into perspective so that their promise does not always entice us into what is wrong? None of these questions has an easy answer. And certainly I have no formula. These are matters of personal decision, decisions dependent on your personal relationship with God and how you think that relationship should be lived out in your choices. My role is to help you identify and define the problem. Then, if you are convinced that you want to do something about the problem, I have a further role. I want to lead you to the revelations of God for the wisdom and strength to find your own answers.

Let's look a bit more closely at the easy choices. They all share an important characteristic: they are *universally without value for the promotion of health.* The best thing that might be said of any of them is that, under ideal circumstances, they are not presently known to be harmful. We're talking about factors that are unnecessary to continued health, about the use of things that, *at the very best,* are harmless.

For example, Paul suggested that Timothy "use a little wine for the sake of your stomach and your frequent ailments" (1 Tim 5:23). I find no convincing scientific evidence, however, that alcohol does anybody any good physically. At best it is merely harmless and, as we have seen, at worst it is a destructive influence of unbelievable proportions. So, somewhere between abstinence and abuse, for most people, there is a level of alcohol intake that can be loosely defined as "moderation." Let's say that you have been able to define that moderation level for yourself and you consume alcohol at that level. What will be your purpose in drinking it? Not to satisfy any basic physiological need because there is none. You drink to satisfy another need that we can broadly define as "pleasure." Is it wrong to seek such pleasure when the substance, at the levels employed, is not known to be harmful?

Most Christians, I suspect, would support the point of view that the ability to enjoy harmless things that give pleasure is a gift of God. But what about things (or amounts) that may be "just a little bit harmful" in transmitting their sensation of pleasure? Do we then make our decisions on the basis of cost versus benefit? Do we say, "If the pleasure is great enough, then it's worth the little bit of harm it may cause"? That, of course, is the kind of logic that temptation feeds on. And temptation is the hazard we always face with choices that have pleasure as their prime goal. Satan loves a compromiser. Pleasure, however it may be defined in specific situations, is his most powerful ammunition for promoting compromise.

So, as we have become more civilized, our opportunities for pleasure have increased—and so have the possibilities that the satisfaction of pleasure will lead to destruction. These include foods that taste good, look good, have good "mouth feel" and are available with minimum inconvenience; substances that calm us down, pep us up or alter our attitudes; things that give us more leisure and require less effort; and decisions that enable us to avoid taking responsibility for our actions.

The choices relating to the satisfaction of these pleasures are, for a growing number of us, life and death decisions. Because of that, you can be assured that Satan will want to participate in those choices with you. If you want to thwart him in that desire, remember that he loves compromise—but he hates commitment.

To establish a life of commitment, we can find no better marching orders than Paul's instructions to the church at Rome: "I appeal to you therefore, brethren, by the mercies of God, to present your bodies as a living sacrifice, holy and acceptable to God, which is your spiritual worship. Do not be conformed to this world but be transformed by the renewal of your mind, that you may prove what is the will of God, what is good and acceptable and perfect" (Rom 12:1-2).

True Christian commitment regards abandonment of simple physical pleasures as a small "sacrifice of the body" to be made in the interest of "spiritual worship." God's acceptance of that sacrifice provides strength to resist conformity, and the power of renewal that makes his will both evident and totally acceptable.

The Promises of God

Why be committed? What do we hope to accomplish by making and keeping commitments? Commitment is our part of an agreement or contract. We enter into the agreement because we are willing to give up something in return for something offered by the other party to the contract. In some cases, the other party may be ourselves.

A New Year's resolution is an example of such an agreement. On New Year's Day you say to yourself, "This year I'm going to start getting more exercise." To which you respond, "Then I will feel better and like myself better." You have made a contract, a commitment in return for a reward. The other party in a commitment agreement can also be another person, as in a marriage. Each partner says to the other, "I will commit myself to you, and you only, for the rest of our days." They have made a contract or covenant of commitment.

If our end of the agreement is *Christian commitment,* God must necessarily be included as a party to the contract. Our part of the bargain is obedience. God's part is his promise to supply the will and strength and grace to make obedience possible. In the first section of this chapter I discussed our obligations to avoid temptation and commit ourselves to "the narrow way." Now I'd like to discuss what God has to tell us about his end of the covenant.

God doesn't expect us to make hard choices by ourselves. In fact, he knows that, if we persist in our claims of self-sufficiency —of independence from his guidance—that we will inevitably make the easy choices and will reap their destructive consequences. Let's say that Jay is forty pounds overweight, and has been for many years. Jay's obesity is becoming more than just a matter of inconvenience and embarrassment. It's beginning to affect his health in significant ways. Jay has tried to lose weight innumerable times. Every diet that comes along is a new challenge, but none of them ever seems to help. Jay may lose a little, temporarily, but always gains it right back. What's his problem? Faulty physiology? Of course not. Jay wants to lose weight without having to make the hard choices. He wants to be thinner, but doesn't want to give up the good life. Jay doesn't have a valid contract; he has made no commitment.

God promises us all of the power and strength necessary to help make hard choices. If Jay wishes, he can draw on that power and strength at any time. To help him develop a perspective on these promises, let's look at what Scripture tells us about them. First, Jesus invites us to share our unbearable burdens with him, and he promises us relief. He says, "Come to me, all who labor and are heavy laden, and I will give you rest. Take my yoke upon you, and learn from me; for I am gentle and lowly in heart, and you will find rest for your souls. For my yoke is easy, and my burden is light" (Mt 11:28-30).

To Jay, and to all the rest of us who are struggling with the temptations of life, Jesus offers an alternative. He promises that he will relieve us of those burdens that we find unbearable. He agrees to take them on himself, to make possible what to us has seemed impossible. But in return he requires that we turn from the good life and commit ourselves to him, that we take on ourselves the easy yoke of dedication to his purposes. He offers an infinite source of strength for dealing with our cares, problems and temptations. All he asks from us in return is commitment to the process, willingness to let go and trust that his power will be sufficient for all our needs.

When Paul was feeling oppressed by the burden of his "thorn in the flesh," he petitioned the Lord three times that it would be taken from him. But his petition was denied. The Lord responded to him, "My grace is sufficient for you, for my power is made perfect in weakness." Trusting in that promise, Paul recommitted himself to his Lord, saying, "I will all the more gladly boast of my weaknesses, that the power of Christ may rest upon me . . . for when I am weak, then I am strong" (2 Cor 12:8-10).

In helping people find the solutions for their own thorns in the flesh—their own physical and emotional weaknesses—I have found three passages from Paul's epistles especially apt. I call them the "all things" lessons. The first I will consider now and the other two later.

In his concluding remarks to the church at Philippi, Paul declared, "I can do *all things* in him who strengthens me" (Phil 4:13). What are the rewards of Christian commitment? The strength and power to do all things. Not just some things, but all things. Most of us, I suspect, never pause to consider the full impact of that statement. By ourselves, we can do nothing—and we are proving it with a failure of self-sufficiency that is destroying our culture with degenerative disease. But, through Christ, all things are possible. We have only to turn to him in trust. He has promised to show us the way.

Christian Decision Making

You have probably been evaluating your own health as you read this book. Perhaps you are not completely satisfied with your stewardship of health or with your prospects for continued good health. Let's assume that my arguments have convinced you that a lifestyle change is the only way you can serve God's purposes— responsibly preserving the health he gave you at birth. In that case, you may be facing the need to abandon a significant portion of the good life. Not just for a couple of days, not just for a few weeks, but for good. That's a substantial commitment—no question about it. And the temptation to avoid it will also be substantial. Look at the record. Inveterate smokers cling to their habit, protesting that they really don't want to live that long anyway. Hard-core diet dropouts find every imaginable excuse not to give up the food habits that keep them fat. And one of the only ways to get a man over fifty to exercise is to wait until he has a heart attack and then make exercise a part of his rehabilitation.

No, these kinds of changes aren't easy. We don't like to give up things we enjoy. We live in a culture that promotes the pursuit of pleasure as a lofty goal. We're admonished to grab all we can, while we can. In such an environment, how do we establish a meaningful commitment to change? At the outset, let's be fully aware that we're dealing with only one fundamental conflict: indulgence in pleasure versus dedication to health. The two are in basic opposition to one another. That is not to say, of course, that a life dedicated to good health has to be a life without pleasure. It just means that you will be establishing a new definition of pleasure, from short-term self-indulgence to long-term well-being and satisfaction. Paul made a clear distinction between the pleasures of the flesh and the joy of life in the Spirit (Rom 8). Commitment to responsible health management represents a quest for a higher order of personal satisfaction. The first step in that quest is to determine which parts of your good life you are prepared to give up in the interest of attaining a higher order of satisfaction.

The next step is to make a commitment, to enter into a covenant or contract for change. A common tendency is to look on such a commitment as a sort of casual exercise in self-denial, to be easily set aside if temptations become too strong. That, of course, is not commitment. It's just fun and games. Lifestyle commitment is a serious agreement to undertake change and, from the outset, to consider such change to be a permanent part of future life. You are wasting your time even considering change unless you are willing to view it from that perspective.

Am I trying to take all of the enjoyment out of your life? No, my intent is exactly the opposite: to help you put *real joy* into your life. Most people have forgotten what it's like to feel really healthy.

For Christians, the decision to change our lifestyles, like all decisions, is one that does not have to be made alone. God has promised to be with us in all of our decisions and to lend his wisdom and guidance to the decision-making process. All we have to do is invite him to participate. I would like to offer some perspectives on making that kind of invitation.

Many of us tend to restrict our efforts to communicate seriously with God to those times when we are confronted with pressing problems—problems whose solutions are beyond our own capabilities. We may be diligent in our table prayers or our evening prayers, seldom missing a day of acknowledging his mighty works. But for those serious invitations for God to come into our lives and take charge, they are probably limited to times of trouble. To make such invitations regular involves two major elements. The first is thanksgiving. The second is subordination.

In his letter to the Ephesians, Paul gave us the starting point for approaching God in prayer, the second of what I call the "all things" lessons. It establishes thanksgiving as an essential element in any invitation for God to be included in our decisions. Paul admonished us to be "giving thanks always for all things unto God and the Father in the name of our Lord Jesus Christ" (Eph 5:20 KJV). Thanksgiving prepares us in two ways to receive and accept God's guidance in making decisions. First, it acknowledges God's supremacy in "all things." It accepts the truth of his responsibility for all we are and all that we hope to be. No matter what our circumstances, no matter how depressing they may appear, always and in everything we have reason to give thanks. Not only do we have the gift of life, but we have it abundantly in all circumstances because Jesus came to be our brother and to set us free from fear and despair. He said to us, "I am with you always, to the close of the age" (Mt 28:20). That fact alone is worthy of our unceasing prayers of thanksgiving.

Second, thanksgiving establishes our willingness to receive

him. When we give thanks we acknowledge God's essential role in giving purpose to our lives. In addition, we acknowledge that no meaningful direction can exist in our lives until his will is made the key factor in our decisions. That acknowledgment then prepares us for the other element of our invitation to God: subordination.

If we intend to invite God to participate in our decisions, we have to subordinate our intellect to his wisdom, our desires to his will. No better example of subordination exists than that of Jesus himself in the Garden of Gethsemane. He was faced with accepting the burden of guilt for the world's disobedience. Praying for relief from that humanly overwhelming burden, Jesus submitted himself to the Father's infinite wisdom and acknowledged, "not as I will, but as thou wilt" (Mt 26:39).

It is folly to invite God to be a part of our decisions in life if we remain unwilling to submit those decisions to him. How do we know what his will is? Where it is not articulated specifically in his Word, he leaves it to our good judgment. However, his purposes for our lives are not that hard to discover. Communication with God is a two-way conversation. If our prayers include some listening, instead of just petitioning, we will find our own judgment in these matters substantially supplemented by the wisdom of God.

Stepping Out in Faith
I would like to use this final spiritual perspective on health first of all as a supplement to the discussion on stress. Then I want to build on this perspective to conclude our study of commitment in personal health management.

Prevention of unwanted stress is not a matter of behavior— it is a matter of faith. It does not result from what you experience —it results from what you believe or don't believe. This point of view is not my own.

Therefore I tell you, do not be anxious about your life, what you shall eat or what you shall drink, nor about your body, what you shall put on. Is not life more than food, and the body more than clothing? Look at the birds of the air: they neither sow nor reap nor gather into barns, and yet your heavenly Father feeds them. Are you not of more value than they? And which of you by being anxious can add one cubit to his span of life? And why are you anxious about clothing? Consider the lilies of the field, how they grow; they neither toil nor spin; yet I tell you, even Solomon in all his glory was not arrayed like one of these. But if God so clothes the grass of the field, which today is alive and tomorrow is thrown into the oven, will he not much more clothe you, *O men of little faith?* (Mt 6:25-30)

Jesus equates anxiety (in our terms, unwanted stress) with having "little faith." What then can we do to strengthen our faith so that unwanted stress can be substantially eliminated? We can start by exploring what faith is. No clearer definition exists than this one: "Now faith is the assurance of things hoped for, the conviction of things not seen" (Heb 11:1).

Uncertainty promotes excess stress. The goal of stress-motivated behavior is to control life events in such a way that all outcomes can be guaranteed—an obviously impossible goal. Nothing in human life is certain. If such efforts are always futile, how do we eliminate uncertainty? Through faith. Life's outcomes don't have to be guaranteed for us to approach life with certainty. We just have to believe that they are certain. That's what faith is: a personal conviction that important outcomes in life, though as yet unseen and without any specific guarantees, will be as hoped for. Faith establishes certainty.

What, then, do we use as the basis for such an assurance, for a faith that puts uncertainty to flight? The promises of God. His Word abounds with guarantees of his willingness—indeed, his

eagerness—to use his mighty resources for us. In him, all outcomes are guaranteed. That truth is beautifully stated in the
third of the "all things" lessons: "We know that in all things God
works for the good of those who love him, who have been called
according to his purpose" (Rom 8:28 NIV).

Faith is the assurance that God's purposes include his specific
concern for me as an individual. Whatever happens, no matter
how incomprehensible at the time, it will accrue to my benefit
and will be underwritten with his unwavering love. Faith is the
conviction that I am indeed created in the image of God and that,
therefore, my identity cannot be diminished by any force on
earth. When I choose to live in that kind of faith, my internal life
will be free of uncertainty. And, without uncertainty, it will be
free of unwanted stress.

Like everything else we've been talking about in these chapters, faith is a choice. For many, it is a difficult choice because
it makes certainty a matter of belief rather than a matter of fact.
Yet it is the only choice that provides anything beyond short-
term rewards.

Faith is the fundamental life choice. Once that choice has
been made, all others become easier. If you want to make a commitment to change, and if you expect the going to be tough, then
a commitment to faith will be the only sure way to success.

Are you having trouble giving up smoking? Have you been trying without success to lose weight? Do you have a high risk for a
heart attack but are unwilling to make the changes that would
lower that risk? Has a false sense of self-sufficiency made you a
prime candidate for some degenerative disease? If so, what are
you going to do about it? Are you ready to commit yourself to a
new lifestyle that can change all of that?

If you are, and are concerned about your ability to keep the
commitment, then I can give you no better advice than to make
faith in God's promises the foundation of your commitment.

With his promises as your standard, you can step out into the realm of "things not seen," assured that God's power can make up for your deficiencies. Trust God that in Christ you can do "all things"—not just some things, but all things—because your faith has equipped you with God's strength. "Have no anxiety about anything, but in everything by prayer and supplication with thanksgiving let your requests be made known to God. And the peace of God, which passes all understanding, will keep your hearts and your minds in Christ Jesus" (Phil 4:6-7).

Appendix
Nutritional Value of
Major Food Groups

In the following table, I have condensed what I consider the most relevant nutritional information for the majority of common foods. Obviously it is impossible to include every different food item consumed. Therefore, I have emphasized foods I would recommend as fundamental to a healthy diet, particularly if the diet is to be restricted in calories.

I have also included a number of food groups that I cannot recommend, but which are major contributors to the average diet. The data on these latter foods are intended to alert you to their nutritional destitution.

To reduce the number of items in the table, I have grouped the foods, as much as possible, by common nutritional content. The calorie data and the assessments of nutritional value are averages for each group. The following information is provided for each food group in the table:

1. Typical serving size.
2. Calories per serving.
3. Percentage of the calories contributed by protein (P), fat (F), carbohydrate (C) and, when applicable, alcohol (A).
4. Examples of foods represented in the group. The listing of examples is not intended to be exhaustive, but rather to provide a basis of identity by which you can add items that are not specifically listed.
5. Assessment of nutritional value. This evaluates individual nutrients

(vitamins, minerals, protein and others) on the basis of their content in the group *per 100 calories consumed,* and assigns one of three ratings on that basis. These ratings are:

Excellent—Contributes more than 20 per cent of the Recommended Dietary Allowance (or reasonable minimum requirement, if no RDA has been established) per 100 calories consumed;

Good—Contributes 15 to 20 per cent of the RDA or minimum requirement per 100 calories;

Fair—Contributes 10 to 15 per cent of the RDA or minimum requirement per 100 calories.

In the case of carbohydrates, nutritional value is based on its established or (most often) estimated tendency to avoid substantial blood-sugar responses. The reason only nine vitamins and minerals are evaluated in this table is that these are the only nutrients for which complete and accurate food content data are currently available. In general, you will find that a diet that is well balanced in these nine nutrients will also provide an adequate supply of the other vitamins and minerals known to be required.

6. Additional comments, when appropriate, on the overall value of the group in responsible human nutrition.

The various food groups in the table are arranged in the following order:

Group Number	Group Name
1-10	Meats, poultry and seafood
11-16	Dairy products and eggs
17-29	Cereal grain products
30-32	Nuts and seeds
33-39	Fruits
40-46	Vegetables
47-51	Sweets
52-59	Miscellaneous

Meats, Poultry and Seafood
Group 1. Lean beef, veal, lamb.
Serving size: 4 oz.
150 calories: 53% P, 47% F, 0% C.
Examples: Rump roast or round steak (trimmed of fat); veal round or leg of lamb; lean ground beef (10% fat).
Good source of protein, phosphorus and vitamin B₃ (niacin). Fair source of iron and potassium.
Group 2. Lean pork.
Serving size: 4 oz.
130 calories: 54% P, 46% F, 0% C.

Examples: Loin roast; shoulder roast; chops or ham (trimmed of fat).
Excellent source of vitamin B_1 (thiamine). Good source of protein and vitamin B_3. Fair source of iron, phosphorus and potassium.
Cured ham provides about 700 mg of sodium per serving.

Group 3. Fat beef.
Serving size: 4 oz.
280 calories: 26% P, 74% F, 0% C.
Examples: Rib roast (untrimmed); regular hamburger (21% fat).
Provides the same nutrients as lean beef but, because of its high fat content, in much lower amounts per calorie consumed.
Not recommended for lower calorie diets.

Group 4. Fat pork.
Serving size: 4 oz.
280 calories: 28% P, 72% F, 0% C.
Examples: Chops or ham (untrimmed).
Provides the same nutrients as lean pork but, because of its high fat content, in much lower amounts per calorie consumed.
Not recommended for lower calorie diets.

Group 5. Liver.
Serving size: 2 oz.
130 calories: 47% P, 47% F, 6% C.
Excellent source of phosphorus, iron, vitamin A, vitamin B_2 (riboflavin) and vitamin B_3. Good source of protein and vitamin C. Fair source of potassium.

Group 6. Specialty meats.
Serving size: as indicated.
130 calories: 18% P, 82% F, 0% C.
Examples: Bacon, 3 slices; pork sausage, 2 oz.; salami, 1 oz.; frankfurter, 1 each.
Of minimum nutritional value.
Not recommended for any but high calorie diets.

Group 7. Fowl.
Serving size: 3 oz.
155 calories: 74% P, 26% F, 0% C.
Examples: Chicken or turkey (baked or boiled, skin removed).
Excellent source of protein, phosphorus and vitamin B_3. Good source of potassium.

Group 8. Fish.
Serving size: as indicated.
140 calories: 66% P, 34% F, 0% C.
Examples: Tuna (canned in water), 4 oz.; salmon, cod, flounder (broiled or baked), 3 oz.
Excellent source of phosphorus. Good source of protein and potassium. Fair source of vitamin B_3.

Group 9. Other seafood I.
Serving size: as indicated.
135 calories: 79% P, 20% F, 1% C.
Examples: Shrimp (boiled), 4 oz.; lobster (boiled), 5 oz.
Good source of protein and phosphorus.

Group 10. Other seafood II.
Serving size: 1/2 cup.
85 calories: 62% P, 24% F, 14% C.
Examples: Oysters or clams.
Excellent source of phosphorus and iron. Good source of protein, calcium, potassium and vitamin B_2. Fair source of vitamins B_1 and B_3.

Dairy Products and Eggs

Group 11. Whole milk.
Serving size: 1 cup.
160 calories: 22% P, 48% F, 30% C.
Excellent source of calcium, phosphorus and vitamin B_2. Good source of potassium. Fair source of protein.
Not recommended for lower calorie diets.

Group 12. Cottage cheese, creamed.
Serving size: 1/2 cup.
120 calories: 53% P, 36% F, 11% C.
Excellent source of phosphorus. Good source of protein and vitamin B_2. Fair source of calcium. Not recommended for lower calorie diets.

Group 13. Low-fat cheese.
Serving size: 1/2 cup.
95 calories: 82% P, 4% F, 14% C.
Examples: Dry-curd cottage cheese; skim-milk cheeses.
Excellent source of protein, phosphorus and vitamin B_2. Good source of calcium.

Group 14. Regular cheese.
Serving size: 1.5 oz.
165 calories: 25% P, 73% F, 2% C.
Examples: Cheddar; Swiss; American.
Excellent source of calcium and phosphorus. Fair source of protein.
Not recommended for lower calorie diets.

Group 15. Other low-fat dairy.
Serving size: 1 cup.
95 calories: 36% P, 11% F, 53% C.
Examples: Skim milk, low-fat yogurt.
Excellent source of calcium, phosphorus, potassium and vitamin B_2. Good source of protein.

Group 16. Eggs.
Serving size: 1 average.
80 calories: 32% P, 65% F, 3% C.
Good source of protein, phosphorus and vitamin A. Fair source of iron and vitamin B_2. Should be limited in lower calorie diets.

Cereal Grain Products
Group 17. Low-fiber bread.
Serving size: as indicated.
85 calories: 10% P, 12% F, 78% C.
Examples: White bread, 1 slice; hamburger or hot dog bun, 1 each; dinner roll, medium, 1 each.
Fair source of carbohydrate and fiber.
Group 18. Medium-fiber bread.
Serving size: 1 slice.
70 calories: 13% P, 11% F, 76% C.
Examples: Cracked wheat or "brown" bread.
Good source of carbohydrate and fiber.
Group 19. High-fiber bread.
Serving size: 1 slice.
75 calories: 16% P, 11% F, 73% C.
Example: Whole-grain bread.
Excellent source of carbohydrate and fiber. Fair source of phosphorus and iron.
Group 20. Ready-to-eat cereal I.
Serving size: 1 cup.
100 calories: 9% P, 3% F, 88% C.
Examples: Corn flakes, wheat flakes (fortified).
Excellent source of the vitamins and minerals used in fortifying (check the label). Good source of carbohydrate and fiber.
Group 21. Ready-to-eat cereal II.
Serving size: 1 cup.
105 calories: 10% P, 4% F, 86% C.
Example: 40% bran flakes (fortified).
Excellent source of carbohydrate and fiber plus the vitamins and minerals used in fortifying (check the label). Good source of phosphorus.
Group 22. Ready-to-eat cereal III.
Serving size: as indicated.
90 calories: 13% P, 5% F, 82% C.
Examples: Puffed wheat or rice (not fortified), 1 1/2 cups; shredded wheat (not fortified), 1 biscuit.
Excellent source of carbohydrate and fiber. Fair source of phosphorus and vitamin B_3.

Group 23. Cooked cereal I.
Serving size: 1 cup
115 calories: 15% P, 5% F, 80% C.
Example: Whole-wheat meal.
Excellent source of carbohydrate and fiber. Good source of phosphorus. Fair source of vitamin B_1.

Group 24. Cooked cereal II.
Serving size: 1 cup.
105 calories: 13% P, 2% F, 86% C.
Example: Farina-style cereal (enriched).
Good source of phosphorus. Fair source of carbohydrate, fiber and vitamin B_1.

Group 25. Pasta.
Serving size: 1 cup.
155 calories: 13% P, 3% F, 84% C.
Examples: Macaroni or spaghetti (enriched).
Fair source of carbohydrate, fiber and vitamin B_1

Group 26. Grain-based snacks.
Serving size: as indicated.
120 calories: 9% P, 30% F, 61% C.
Examples: Saltine crackers, 10 each; 3-ring pretzels, 10 each; 1-inch square cheese crackers, 24 each. Of minimal nutritional value.

Group 27. Popcorn (dry-popped).
Serving size: 4 cups.
90 calories: 13% P, 11% F, 86% C.
Excellent source of carbohydrate and fiber. Fair source of phosphorus.

Group 28. Pancakes/waffles.
Serving size: as indicated.
125 calories: 13% P, 30% F, 57% C.
Examples: Pancakes, 4-inch diameter, 2 each; waffle, 1 large.
Fair source of carbohydrate and phosphorus.

Group 29. Rice/corn.
Serving size: as indicated.
140 calories: 9% P, 4% F, 87% C.
Examples: Brown rice (unpolished), 2/3 cup; white rice, 3/4 cup; whole-kernel corn, 1 cup.
Excellent source of carbohydrate and fiber (except white rice, which is only a fair source of both).

Nuts and Seeds
Group 30. Peanuts.
Serving size: as indicated.
175 calories: 16% P, 72% F, 12% C.

Examples: Peanuts, 1 oz.; peanut butter (natural), 2 tbsp.
Good source of fiber and vitamin B₃. Fair source of phosphorus.
Because of their high fat content, not recommended for lower calorie diets.

Group 31. Other nuts.
Serving size: 1 oz.
185 calories: 7% P, 84% F, 9% C.
Examples: Walnuts; pecans; Brazil nuts; almonds.
Good source of fiber (especially almonds).
Their very high fat content makes them undesirable for lower calorie diets.

Group 32. Seeds.
Serving size: 1 oz.
160 calories: 16% P, 71% F, 13% C.
Example: Sunflower seeds.
Excellent source of fiber, phosphorus and vitamin B_1. Fair source of iron and potassium.
Their very high fat content limits their usefulness in lower calorie diets.

Fruits
Group 33. Citrus fruits/juice.
Serving size: as indicated.
90 calories: 6% P, 2% F, 92% C.
Examples: Orange, 1 large; orange juice (fresh or reconst. frozen), 3/4 cup; grapefruit (unsweetened), 1 cup sections; grapefruit juice (unsweetened), 1 cup.
Excellent source of potassium and vitamin C. Fair source of vitamin B_1.

Group 34. Other fruit I.
Serving size: as indicated.
95 calories: 4% P, 6% F, 90% C.
Examples: Apple, 1 medium; apple juice, 3/4 cup; apple sauce (unsweetened), 1 cup; pear, 1 medium; cherries (unsweetened), 1 cup.
Good source of carbohydrate and potassium. Fair source of fiber.

Group 35. Other fruit II.
Serving size: as indicated.
105 calories: 6% P, 10% F, 84% C.
Examples: Strawberries, 2 cups; blackberries/raspberries, 1 cup; blueberries, 1 cup.
Excellent source of vitamin C and fiber. Good source of iron and potassium. Fair source of carbohydrate.

Group 36. Other fruit III.
Serving size: as indicated.
85 calories: 7% P, 3% F, 90% C.
Examples: Peach, 1 medium; cantaloupe, 1/2 of a 5-inch diameter; apricots

(12 per pound), 5 each.

Excellent source of potassium, vitamin A and vitamin C. Fair source of iron.

Group 37. Other fruit IV.

Serving size: as indicated.

100 calories: 4% P, 2% F, 94% C.

Examples: Banana, 1 medium; plums, 2 1/3 inch diameter, 3 each.

Excellent source of potassium. Fair source of carbohydrate.

Group 38. Dried fruit.

Serving size: as indicated.

105 calories: 3% P, 1% F, 96% C.

Examples: Apricots, 8 large halves; dates, 4 large; prunes, 4 medium; raisins, 1/4 cup.

Excellent source of potassium and fiber. Good source of carbohydrate. Fair source of iron.

Group 39. Fruit canned in syrup.

Serving size: 1/2 cup.

95 calories: 2% P, 1% F, 97% C.

Examples: Fruit cocktail; peaches; pears; pineapple.

Of virtually no significant nutritional value. Predominantly sugar.

Vegetables

Group 40. Potato.

Serving size: 1 large.

145 calories: 11% P, 1% F, 88% C.

Excellent source of potassium and vitamin C. Fair source of carbohydrate, phosphorus, vitamin B_3 and fiber.

Group 41. Beans.

Serving size: 2/3 cup.

150 calories: 26% P, 4% F, 70% C.

Examples: Navy, kidney, lima beans.

Excellent source of potassium, carbohydrate and fiber. Good source of phosphorus and iron. Fair source of protein.

Group 42. Yellow vegetables.

Serving size: as indicated.

95 calories: 8% P, 5% F, 87% C.

Examples: Carrots, cooked, 2 cups; pumpkin, cooked, 1 cup; winter squash, cooked, 1 cup.

Excellent source of potassium and vitamin A. Good source of vitamin C. Fair source of carbohydrate and fiber.

Group 43. Dark green vegetables.

Serving size: as indicated.

50 calories: 35% P, 12% F, 53% C.

Examples: Broccoli, cooked, 1 1/4 cup; romaine lettuce, chopped, 5 cups; collard greens, cooked, 3/4 cup; spinach, cooked, 1 cup; spinach, raw, chopped, 3 cups.

Excellent source of calcium, phosphorus, iron, potassium, vitamin A, vitamin B_2, vitamin C and fiber. Good source of carbohydrate. Fair source of protein, vitamin B_1 and vitamin B_3. Per calorie, the best source of overall nutrition available. (Popeye wasn't fooling.)

Group 44. Other vegetables I.
Serving size: as indicated.
50 calories: 19% P, 5% F, 76% C.

Examples: Tomatoes, raw, 2 medium; tomatoes, canned, 1 cup; tomato juice, 1 cup; green beans or asparagus, cooked, 1 1/2 cup; zucchini, chopped, raw or cooked, 2 cups.

Excellent source of iron, potassium, vitamin A, vitamin B_1, and vitamin C. Good source of carbohydrate, fiber, phosphorus and vitamin B_3. Fair source of vitamin B_2.

Group 45. Other vegetables II.
Serving size: as indicated.
20 calories: 19% P, 7% F, 74% C.

Examples: Cabbage, shredded, raw, 1 cup; head lettuce, chopped, 2 cups; cucumber, chopped, 1 cup; cauliflower, chopped, raw or cooked, 1 cup; celery, chopped, 1 cup; eggplant, chopped, 1/2 cup.

Excellent source of phosphorus, potassium and vitamin C. Good source of carbohydrate, fiber, calcium, iron, vitamin B_1 and vitamin B_2. Fair source of vitamin B_3.

Group 46. Frozen peas.
Serving size: 1/2 cup.
60 calories: 29% P, 4% F, 67% C.

Example: Green peas, frozen, cooked.

Excellent source of phosphorus, potassium, vitamin B_1, vitamin B_3, vitamin C and fiber. Good source of carbohydrate, iron and vitamin A. Fair source of protein and vitamin B_2.

Sweets
Group 47. Candy.
Serving size: 1 oz.
125 calories: 7% P, 42% F, 51% C.

Examples: Fudge with nuts; peanut bar; vanilla creams.
Almost exclusively fat and sugar. Of no nutritional value.

Group 48. Pastries.
Serving size: as indicated.
310 calories: 5% P, 46% F, 49% C.

Examples: Cake with icing, 1 medium slice; pie (apple, custard, pecan, lemon), 1 medium slice; danish pastry, 1 large; doughnut, 1 large; eclair, 1 average. Predominantly fat and sugar. Of no nutritional value.

Group 49. Ice cream.
Serving size: 1 cup.
255 calories: 9% P, 49% F, 42% C.
Example: Regular commercial ice cream.
Fair source of calcium.
Little additional nutritional value because of high fat and sugar content. (Note: Rich ice cream and frozen custard are about 30% higher in calories for the same serving size.)

Group 50. Gelatin dessert.
Serving size: 1 cup.
160 calories: 7% P, 1% F, 92% C.
Little nutritional value per calorie consumed because of the high sugar content.

Group 51. Sugar-sweetened soft drinks.
Serving size: 12 fl. oz.
145 calories: 0% P, 0% F, 100% C.
Examples: Soda pop; most canned fruit drinks; most dry drink mixes, including breakfast mixes.
Of no significant nutritional value (even if they contain added vitamin C) because of their high sugar content.

Miscellaneous

Group 52. Tomato-based sauce.
Serving size: 1/4 cup.
50 calories: 10% P, 24% F, 66% C.
Example: Spaghetti sauce without meat.
Excellent source of potassium and vitamin A. Good source of vitamin C. Fair source of carbohydrate and fiber.
Catsup is proportionately less nutritious because of its generous sugar content.

Group 53. Meat gravy.
Serving size: 1/4 cup.
165 calories: 3% P, 77% F, 20% C.
Of minimum nutritional value because of its high fat content.

Group 54. Salad dressing, regular.
Serving size: 1 tbsp.
85 calories: 0% P, 98% F, 2 % C.
Examples: Roquefort; French; Italian; mayonnaise; Thousand Island.
Of no nutritional value. Almost all fat.

Group 55. Salad dressing, diet.
Serving size: 1 tbsp.

15 calories: 0% P, 82% F, 18% C.

Examples: Roquefort; French; Italian; Thousand Island.

Of no nutritional value but the total calorie cost is low.

Group 56. Butter/margarine.

Serving size: 1 tsp.

35 calories: 0% P, 100% F, 0% C.

Fair source of vitamin A. Not recommended for lower calorie diets.

Group 57. Pizza.

Serving size: 1/7 of a 10-inch pizza.

155 calories: 20% P, 32% F, 48% C.

Example: Plain cheese pizza.

Fair source of carbohydrate, calcium and phosphorus.

Not recommended for lower calorie diets.

Group 58. Beer, regular.

Serving size: 12 fl. oz.

150 calories: 3% P, 0% F, 36% C, 61% A.

Fair source of phosphorus and vitamin B₃.

Of minimum nutritional value because of the high calorie contribution from alcohol.

Group 59. Other alcoholic beverage.

Serving size: as indicated.

110 calories: 0% P, 0% F, 16% C, 84% A.

Examples: Table wines, 4 fl. oz.; Manhattan, martini or old fashioned, 2 fl. oz.; 90-proof liquor in a typical mixed drink, 1 to 1 1/2 fl. oz.

Of no nutritional value.

Notes

Chapter 1: Life, Death and the Perils of Progress
[1]The historical statistics quoted in this chapter come primarily from a two-volume compilation issued in 1975 by the United States Bureau of the Census, entitled *Historical Statistics of the United States, Colonial Times to 1970.*
[2]In addition to specific references which will be cited later, data on the current state of health of the American population were obtained from among the following government publications:

Baselines for Setting Health Goals and Standards, Department of Health, Education and Welfare (DHEW) Publ. No. (HRA) 77-640.

Facts of Life and Death, DHEW Publ. No. (PHS) 79-1222.

Healthy People, DHEW Publ. No. (PHS) 79-55071.

Health in the United States, DHEW Publ. No. (PHS) 80-1233.

[3]Richard B. Singer and Louis Levinson, eds., *Medical Risks: Patterns of Mortality and Survival* (Lexington, Mass.: Lexington Books, 1976), p. 167. This is a reference volume sponsored by the Association of Life Insurance Medical Directors of America and the Society of Actuaries.

Chapter 2: Making Choices
[1]*Historical Statistics of the United States.*
[2]*Obesity in America,* National Institutes of Health (NIH) Publ. No. 80-359.
[3]*Alcohol and Health,* Department of Health and Human Services (DHHS) Publ. No. (ADM) 81-1080.

Chapter 4: Nutrition, Health and Disease

[1]*Obesity in America.*

[2]M. J. Perley and D. M. Kipnis, "Plasma Insulin Responses to Oral and Intravenous Glucose: Studies in Normal and Diabetic Subjects," *Journal of Clinical Investigation* 46 (1967):1954.

[3]*Primary Prevention of Atherosclerotic Diseases,* rev. April 1972. This is a report of the Inter-Society Commission for Heart Disease Resources, New York. *Dietary Goals for the United States,* 2d ed. (1977). This is a report of the Select Committee on Nutrition and Human Needs, United States Senate.

[4]*Dietary Goals for the United States.*

[5]The history of research on the possible role of diet (and especially sugar) in the cause of CVD has been reviewed in detail by R. A. Ahrens, "Sucrose, Hypertension and Heart Disease: An Historical Perspective," *American Journal of Clinical Nutrition* 24 (1974):403.

[6]F. Dreyfuss, "The Incidence of Myocardial Infarctions in Various Communities in Israel," *American Heart Journal,* 45 (1953):749; A. Cohen et al., "Involuntary Sclerosis and Diastolic Hypertension," *The Lancet* 2 (1960):1050.

[7]A. Cohen et al., "Change of Diet of Yemenite Jews in Relation to Diabetes and Ischemic Heart Disease," *The Lancet* 2 (1961):1399.

[8]A. Cohen, "Prevalence of Diabetes among Different Ethnic Jewish Groups in Israel," *Metabolism* 10 (1961):50.

[9]J. D. Abernathy, "Sodium and Potassium in High Blood Pressure," *Food Technology,* December 1979, p. 57.

[10]N. Simpson, "Diabetes in Families of Diabetics," *The Canadian Medical Association Journal* 98 (1968):427. A. Cohen, "Prevalence of Diabetes."

[11]A. Cohen, "Prevalence of Diabetes."

[12]A. Cohen et al., "Change of Diet of Yemenite Jews."

[13]G. D. Campbell et al., "Sugar Intake and Diabetics," *Diabetes* 16 (1967):62.

[14]*The Sweetener Report,* published in *Food Engineering* (July 1982, p. 75) estimates the 1983 per capita consumption of nutritive sweeteners (sugar and corn syrups) at 127 pounds per year—or about 632 calories per day. The U.S. Department of Agriculture estimates the average total per capita calorie consumption at about 2,900 calories per day. Thus, sugar and syrup consumption currently constitute almost 22 per cent of total average calorie intake for the American people.

[15]*Historical Statistics of the United States.*

[16]Perley and Kipnis, "Plasma Insulin Responses."

[17]*Diabetes Data,* DHEW Publ. No. (NIH) 78-1468.

[18]Perley and Kipnis, "Plasma Insulin Responses."

[19]*Heart Facts* (American Heart Association, 1984). *Diabetes Data.*

[20]E. A. Nikkila et al., "Plasma-Insulin in Coronary Heart Disease," *The Lancet* 1 (1965):508.

[21]Much of the best work on the role of fiber in the prevention of lower bowel disease has been done by Dr. Denis Burkitt, a British physician whose research career spans decades and continents in scope. Dr. Burkitt's popular book on the subject is an excellent presentation in everyday terms and provides a thorough bibliography of relevant literature: *Eat Right— To Stay Healthy and Enjoy Life More* (New York: Arco Publishing Co., 1979).

Chapter 5: Eating to Stay Well

[1]For those who are interested in a more detailed discussion of dietary needs and allowances, I recommend a comprehensive yet inexpensive book published by the National Academy of Sciences. Called *Recommended Dietary Allowances,* this book is a study report from the Academy's Food and Nutrition Board. It compiles the most recent information from the scientific literature on the nutritional needs of the human body. This study is the basis for the so-called RDAs (Recommended Daily Allowance). The report reviews over 700 scientific sources and is unquestionably the most authoritative document currently available on the subject. This information is updated every five years. The Ninth Edition, published in 1980, is presently available from: Office of Publications, National Academy of Sciences, 2101 Constitution Ave., Washington, DC 20418.

[2]*The Sweetener Report.*

[3]All of the data on the nutritive value of common food items were obtained from the U.S. Department of Agriculture publication, *Nutritive Value of American Foods* (Agriculture Handbook No. 456, November 1975).

[4]*Nutritive Value of Convenience Foods,* 3d ed., compiled by West Suburban Dietetic Association (Hines, Ill.: 1982).

[5]J. D. Abernathy, "Sodium and Potassium in High Blood Pressure."

Chapter 6: Alcohol, Tobacco, Caffeine

[1]*Alcohol and Health.*

[2]*Historical Statistics of the United States.*

[3]*Cancer Facts and Figures* (American Cancer Society, 1983).

[4]*Heart Facts.*

[5]*Why People Smoke Cigarettes,* Public Health Service (PHS) Publ. No. (PHS) 83-50195.

[6]H. Steinberg, ed., *Scientific Basis of Drug Dependence* (New York: Grune & Stratton, 1969), pp. 5ff.

[7]F. H. Meyers et al., *Review of Medical Pharmacology,* 5th ed. (Los Altos, Calif.: Lange Medical Publications, 1968), pp. 120ff.

[8]B. A. Kihlman, *Caffeine and Chromosomes* (Amsterdam: Elsevier Press, 1977), pp. 11ff.

Chapter 8: Stress

[1]A. C. Guyton, *Basic Human Physiology: Normal Function and Mechanisms of Disease,* 2d ed. (Philadelphia: Saunders, 1977), p. 600.

[2]J. C. Buell, and R. S. Eliot, "Psychosocial and Behavioral Influences in the Pathogenesis of Acquired Cardiovascular Disease," *American Heart Journal* 100 (1980):723.

[3]T. H. Holmes, and R. H. Rahe, "The Social Readjustment Rating Scale," *Psychomatic Research* 11 (1967):213.

Chapter 9: Spiritual Perspectives on Staying Well

[1]C. S. Lewis, *Screwtape Letters* (New York: Macmillan, 1961), p. 89.